breathe, little boy, breathe!

BREATHE, LITTLE BOY, BREATHE!

an emergency room doctor's story
Stephen B. Seager, M.D.

Prentice-Hall, Inc., Englewood Cliffs, New Jersey 07632

Breathe, Little Boy, Breathe! An
Emergency Room Doctor's Story
by Stephen B. Seager, M.D.

Copyright © 1981 by Stephen B. Seager, M.D.

Address inquiries to Prentice-Hall, Inc.,
Englewood Cliffs, N.J. 07632
Printed in the United States of America
Prentice-Hall International, Inc., London
Prentice-Hall of Australia, Pty. Ltd., Sydney
Prentice-Hall of Canada, Ltd., Toronto
Prentice-Hall of India Private Ltd., New Delhi
Prentice-Hall of Japan, Inc., Tokyo
Prentice-Hall of Southeast Asia Pte. Ltd., Singapore
Whitehall Books Limited, Wellington, New Zealand
10 9 8 7 6 5 4 3 2 1

Library of Congress Cataloging in Publication Data

Seager, Stephen B.
    Breathe, little boy, breathe!

    1. Hospitals—Emergency service. 2. Hospitals—
United States—Emergency service. 3. Seager, Stephen B.
4. Emergency physicians—United States—Biography.
    I. Title.
RA975.5.E5S43   616'.025'0924   81-4656
ISBN 0-13-081729-5   AACR2

To the people of Philadelphia and of Phoenix, my once and future patients.

To Dr. Michael Krentz, who hired a young inexperienced doctor and stuck with him.

To my parents, my sister Nancy, and my children, Brett, Shannan, and Stephen. I love you dearly.

But mainly to my wife Sandy, whom I love most of all.

part one

SATUR-DAY NIGHT

1.

"The man in bed one is dead," the departing doctor said in a rote monotone. "An old alcoholic, probably penetrated an ulcer or ruptured a varix. He bled out right quick. The mortuary has been called," he added. Speedy removal of the body was essential. It lay in a much needed bed. There were other, live, people waiting.

"Bed two has just arrived," he went on, shuffling the first chart beneath a pile of others. "I glanced at him briefly. It looks like pulmonary edema. I'd check him first." I looked up. The patient had been connected to oxygen and wired on a monitor. A nurse stabbed his arm with an intravenous line.

"Bed three is an elbow... kid fell roller skating. He's down in X-ray.

"Bed four is an appendix... surgeon on the way." He slid another chart beneath the rotating pile. "She should be in the O.R. within the hour.

"Bed five is a man with abdominal pain. He has lab work and X-rays pending.

"Bed six is going home, sore throat.

"Bed seven is a broken hip waiting for a room."

With the required recitation at an end he smiled, probably for the first time in hours. His shift was over. He was going home. He looked like a man being discharged from the army.

"Have a nice night," he said with a relieved sigh and left. Left me with the stack of charts. And the patients. It was 7:10.

Mr. Barnes, the man in bed two, was indeed, as my predecessor had suggested, in pulmonary edema. Fluid was filling his lungs because his heart was not working right. He had,

I learned later, been getting slowly worse for two weeks but had refused to see a doctor. Then he coughed blood on his wife's new carpet. Enough was enough. He was taken to the hospital.

I hadn't mentioned it to the previous doctor, as he had been so anxious to leave, but I had seen these people before. The same thin, panting man and his rippling, obese wife had passed me in the parking lot.

She had emerged from the passenger side of an older model car, the kind with fins for fenders, catching her porcine hip on the door handle. Waddling around the front of the auto, dimming both headlights with her voluminous frame, she had gruffly extracted a small, wispish man from the driver's side. As parents do with a fallen child, she had brushed him off and stood him straight. He teetered for a moment but, with her firmly grasping an elbow, they had made for the hospital entrance.

I should have helped the pair but didn't. I stood like an audience, watching the action before me. I watched the woman adjust her winged glasses and tug on droopy pants; her hair was in curlers, with one dangling roller spilling tangled ends of wet hair. I watched the spindly man shuffle along the macadam drive, his slippers making a scuffing noise, like paper over wood. I heard their voices. Hers, strong and forceful. His, faint and threadlike. I heard his labored breathing.

They were the same sounds, her voice and his breathing, that I now heard as I met them again. This time he was upright in bed and she was seated beside him. Even as he fought for breath, his wife continued to nag. How was she to clean the mess on the carpet? Her husband was respiring too rapidly to answer. "And it was a brand new carpet!" she added, slapping the bedrail.

Over the course of an hour the crisis passed. With the aid of medication and a breathing treatment, Mr. Barnes began to pink up. He puffed more easily. The catheter that collected his urine brimmed with clear, fresh fluid. We had successfully drained both the man's soggy lungs through his bladder.

He survived the evening, although, most likely, neither

4

he nor his wife would have minded very much had he died. But he was not going to do that. Not tonight. Not on my shift.

A stable Mr. Barnes was transferred to the Coronary Care Unit. While he was being wheeled away, lights flashing and tubes flushing, the obese woman's tirade continued. Now she was gesturing with her hands. Certain that he would live, she had forgotten about the rug. "How could you put me through this!" she shouted as they were lost through a swinging door. "You nearly scared me to death!" The transporting orderly, last to leave, gave us a smile.

Quickly I rid myself of all minor problems. The appendix case was sent upstairs for surgery. The roller skater's elbow was cast and sent home. The sore throat was cultured, treated, and released. The broken hip was dispatched to the first available room. The body in bed one, like a sausage, was encased in a bag and taken away. All this was simple. The fellow in bed five, the man with the abdominal pain, whose lab and X-rays were pending, proved not to be so simple.

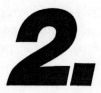
2.

LaVar Erickson had walked into the Emergency Room. He never walked out. That evening he had experienced slight stomach pains. Lying down did not bring relief, as someone had suggested; nor did Alka-Seltzer, his own favorite remedy, seem to help.

He had been attending a large family reunion over which he was presiding patriarch, and thus he had received much attention and advice regarding his developing malady. Although the consensus was "nothing serious," a more conservative wing held sway and it was decided to come to the hospital, "just to be sure."

Most of the Erickson descendants accompanied their progenitor to the Emergency Room. Among them were his wife, brothers and sisters, assorted spouses, his children with their children, and I believe, a neighbor. I remember them all because I met them—after Mr. Erickson died.

What had begun as an upset stomach was now a constant ache. I parted the curtain behind which he and his wife sat, and spoke to them both. During my examination (I always recheck any patients left from the previous shift) I elicited, from a gentle stomach poke, more response than anticipated. Before I left, this increased pain was mentioned by both him and his wife. I expressed my sympathy, which was real, but related to them that I could do nothing about relief until I was absolutely certain about the cause of the pain. And I would not be certain until his lab results and X-rays were back. I added, as small consolation, that the blood had already been drawn and he was next to go for X-rays. It would be just a little while longer, I told them. Then I left.

I don't like to see people suffer, but in the case of abdominal pain, as any doctor will tell you, there is no other choice. Painkillers mask pain, and pain is a crucial symptom, my only barometer of a condition's progress. Without an accurate assessment of pain I cannot judge correctly. And, despite suffering, I must do this.

Once back in the nursing station, I pulled the correct chart before me and began to record my findings. This done, I glanced at the name. It was then that I realized I did not know what the Ericksons looked like. I remembered the man's stomach. I could recall his wife's voice, short and anxious, while depicting her husband's pain. But I could not recreate either face. Had I been called upon to describe the couple, I could not have done so. This, however, was to change with my next visit, when I would deliver the first blast of bad news. Then I would notice every fleck in their eyes and wrinkle in their clothing.

Tired from writing, I turned and gazed out into the hall. I saw a young boy pass with one hand wrapped in a towel. A slow trickle of blood dripped to the floor. He looked like Hansel leaving a trail of blood crumbs. He wasn't crying, as I might have expected, but instead only looked embarrassed. His father, walking but a step behind, seemed more angry than concerned. I knew there was a good story behind all this. And I would have heard that story were it not for the man who crashed in his hang glider.

The boy with the bloody towel stepped nimbly aside, as did his irate father, out of the path of a careening gurney. A man was splayed like a wounded animal across the rocketing cart. Two paramedics were furiously pounding his shirtless chest. His pants were shredded. What once had been a face was now a bubbling mass of crimson fluid, embedded with dirt. I knew it was his face only because there were feet at the other end.

One shoulder had been pushed up as if a large rock were buried underneath. From his right thigh a steepled spike of shredded bone stuck into the air. I was careful not to graze the orthous spicule; I would have received a nasty cut. Some tremendous force had split this person's femur and pushed it out through the skin.

In one motion the contorted mass was thrown from the cart onto a bed. Nurses, like angry bees, collected and hovered while attaching strands of equipment.

I fought a curious crowd, they too having been attracted by the uproar, and at last touched bedside. I surveyed the human carnage. Initially I wondered why a breathing tube had not been inserted into the man's trachea. This was standard procedure in any such situation, airway maintenance being the first priority. Then I saw why. The man's mouth, located only with difficulty, was full of metal. An initial cursory inspection showed the obstruction to be some sort of mechanical device. A control box, I found out later, was trapped behind a row of broken teeth.

With the aid of a nurse, the twisted wreckage was removed. This broke any remaining teeth. Once it was out, blood gushed in its wake. Forceful suction quickly scoured away the gurgling effluent and revealed a throat. I pushed a tube in and attached a balloon bag.

It took but three pumps of the bag to end our efforts. It became obvious from those few blasts of air that this man's problems, no matter what they ultimately proved to be, were incompatible with life. I ordered everyone away and removed the air-giving tube, setting it next to the mouth box which lay beside him. Blood dripped from both into a red, ever widening circle.

When the breathing bag had been compressed, forcing air down the tube, toward the man's lungs, the air came back—but it had not come back out the tube. Once pumped, the air had taken a circuitous route and, like a surfacing whale, spouted out a closed eye. It lifted the eyelid and hissed. Like a calliope. Opening the lid revealed the entire eyeball to be gone.

The metal in the man's mouth turned out to be the control for a motorized hang glider. Apparently the pilot was to hold the kite with both hands and maneuver it with a stick clenched between his teeth. Somehow this man's teeth had driven him into the side of a mountain, which had crammed the control box down his throat, and broken every bone in his body. And it made air come out his eye. The mortuary was called again. He was twenty-three.

Then I remembered the hand. I remembered because I heard the father once again chiding his son. From the next bed I could see feet pacing beneath the drawn curtain.

I asked a nurse if she would have the berating man step out while I checked the boy. She spoke to him and he left, but only after shooting one last verbal salvo while rounding the corner.

The son was dejectedly sitting on the edge of the bed. His chart said fourteen but he looked younger. Eleven would have been a good guess.

"What happened to you?" I asked in a noncommital manner, hiding an intense curiosity.

"I sort of stabbed my hand," the boy replied sheepishly.

"I see," I said, and removed the towel that had been wrapped around his hand since I first saw him.

Piercing the young man's hand was an intact hunting knife. One half showed through the palm side and one half through the knuckle side. It was buried up to the hilt.

I have learned from other, similar situations not to make witty or sharp remarks at times like these, despite what, at the moment, is an overwhelming urge. I have trained myself to remain poker faced and to ask nothing but the pertinent questions.

"Why did you stab your hand?"

"It's a long story."

"I've got time."

I didn't but planned on making some.

"Well you see, my friend and I were sort of trying to impress this girl we know," the boy began in the shy way that young men do when discussing the opposite sex, "by doing a circus trick that we saw on TV. Anyway, we wanted to show this girl, a friend of ours, that we could do it too."

"And you got to be the victim?"

"Yeah, my friend said that he had read in a magazine somewhere about throwing knives and knew how to do it."

"He didn't know," I said looking down again at the impaled hand.

"It would seem that way," the boy replied.

"Your father is pretty mad, I guess," I said, stating the obvious.

"He sure is," the lad said with a sigh. "We used our living room painting for a background."

I placed his hand on a pillow and called our hand surgeon. That night the boy would have the Bowie knife removed. I don't know if anyone ever fixed the painting.

3.

There is a sign posted in the Emergency Room window, a Xerox copy pasted to the glass, which depicts a hand-drawn Charlie Brown. He is dressed in a dark, three-piece suit and looks forlornly at Lucy. He says, "Doing a good job in the E.R. is like wetting your pants in a black suit. It gives you a warm feeling but no one notices."

The sign is right. Those for whom you do the most know the least. The effusive thanks and accolades come from treatment of the small items, sore throats, sprained ankles, and stitched lacerations, things requiring minimum expertise to which the general public can relate. The real lifesavers, the lightning fast decisions or perfect drug concoctions, usually pass without notice. Those most desperately ill, whose ultimate course is reversed, literally turned from death back to life, are rapidly whisked to the Intensive Care Unit, there to awaken and heap praise upon that staff. Because of a coma or concussion, they are never certain if they were even in the Emergency Room.

Perhaps the E.R. events are too unfamiliar, too momentous, too rapid, or just too overwhelming to appreciate. Whatever the reason, it happens often, and it wears you down. Mr. Cohen had this problem. He couldn't relate. His bout with hypoglycemia was something that was too large to understand and went by too swiftly.

Abraham Cohen was literally dragged in by his family, their arms beneath his shoulders, and laid on our front landing. The weight of his body triggered the electric doors. A son, one of the draggers, leaned in and asked for help. Someone else cradled the old man's head. Our startled receptionist leaped and ran for the door. She took one look at the supine man and his excited entourage, then ran back inside. She returned with two technicians and a nurse. The three quickly scooped the gentleman onto a cart and, followed by the family, maneuvered him inside. While the receptionist stood on the ramp to catch her breath, she noticed that there was no car nearby. She looked out into the lot where the Cohens might have parked their car. An overhead sign read "Ambulances only." The family must have seen the sign, she told me later, parked below and hauled their father, like a bag of corn, across the pavement, up the incline, and to the door.

I watched the flurry go by. The retrieving staff and their cart-borne cargo noisily hustled into the Code Room, a special area, closed off from the rest of the E.R., where particularly critical cases are handled. Anyone in this room receives priority attention. It is stocked and ready for immediate action. And this is precisely what Mr. Cohen required. I trotted in behind the group.

The man's face was dusky, the color of a near-dead sunset. He had barely perceptible pulses and no spontaneous breathing. His blood pressure was 0/0.

"Do we have any history on this man?" I asked as a short plastic tube was inserted into his mouth and the breather attached. Pumping began on his chest. To facilitate heart monitor lead placement, his shirt was cut away. In an instant a large-bore intravenous line was inserted in his arm.

"No, no history," a nurse replied. She was the one who had assisted in bringing the patient. "But I'll run out and see if he has a wife with him. I'll talk to her." With that, she was gone. Another nurse stepped in.

"Give him two amps of Narcan, I.V. push, followed by an amp of fifty percent glucose," I said while reading a paper strip from the EKG machine. Then I checked the man's sluggish pupils.

The medications were drawn. The first, Narcan, is used to counteract narcotic overdosage, not at all uncommon in older folks. Most people imagine the drug problem is restricted to young abusers, but this is not so. There are as many, if not more, elderly addicts, usually people afflicted with a painful chronic ailment who have slowly become dependent upon pain medication and who continue its use after the original complaint's successful resolution. Drugs then are a prime consideration in patients who are comatose, regardless of age.

The second drug, glucose, or sugar, will reverse hypoglycemia, low blood sugar. While most people who claim to suffer from hypoglycemia really do not, those who do may experience life-threatening episodes of illness. A low blood sugar problem is corrected by simply giving sugar, and since diabetes, which can produce low as well as high blood sugar, is very common, I always check for this too. Blood was drawn for the lab and the medicines given.

Narcan did nothing. Chest compression and artificial respiration still had to be used to keep Mr. Cohen alive. But it was different with the sugar. Barely one minute after its administration, his pulse began to quicken and firm. Gasps erupted from silence. Pupils contracted and eyes opened. Another slug of sugar was given and a continuous drip begun. Within five minutes the man was awake and talking. We had discovered a new diabetic.

"I told you I wanted Term," the newly revived man said looking around, somewhat puzzled. He was still lying flat but had raised his head. "I said I wanted the Term Policy and you bought Whole Life!" he continued.

Two startled nurses exchanged raised-eyebrow glances.

"And from your cousin the crook, no less," Mr. Cohen went on, "I can't believe it. That man has never done an honest day's work in his life, and he talked you into Whole Life insurance!" Again the old man gazed about. He shook his head, leaned up on an elbow, and honed in on one particular nurse. "You're not Irene!" he said, nonplussed. Then he patted his chest. "Where are my glasses?" he shouted angrily. Confusion was mounting. He tugged at the wires connecting his chest to our heart machine. "Where is my shirt?" he yelled. His shredded garment and bifocals were passed to him from a nearby counter. Mr. Cohen removed the spectacles from a brown case hooking the prongs around his ears. Then he held up the ripped shirt. Dozens of tiny cloth flags waved as he brushed them with his hand.

"Where the hell am I?" he stammered quietly. "And where is Irene?"

Suddenly the door opened and a woman appeared, escorted in by the nurse who had gone to the lobby seeking relatives. "Are you all right, Abe?" the old woman asked as her head turned toward the beeping machines and blinking lights. She stepped back. The nurse assured her it was okay and nudged the lady forward. She took small, timid steps to the bedside.

Her husband had lain back. He was staring straight up, no doubt wondering why the living room ceiling had changed color.

"Are you all right, Abe?" the shy lady repeated a bit more loudly. "We were all so worried."

At the sound of a familiar voice Abraham Cohen sat up. The threads of former conversation were connected again.

"Worried?" the sitting man said, forgetting his unusual surroundings. "Worried? If I were you, the only thing I would be worried about is your cousin the insurance salesman. The nogoodnik. And from him you bought a policy!" He again went down. "Oy," he moaned, "and Whole Life no less, at our age."

"I didn't think you would mind, Abe," the smallish woman said, peering nervously from side to side. She hoped no one was listening to their quarrel, the quarrel that had begun at home but had been interrupted. "You are always saying that we need to save a little money. And who can have enough insurance?" Her words had the sound of an oft repeated phrase, as if she were parroting her cousin.

"But Irene," the befuddled man said again, still looking straight up, a palm now placed directly over his forehead, "why from your cousin? Why from the gonif?"

Hypoglycemia does this. It's like anesthesia: you forget. When your brain doesn't get enough sugar, it clicks off. Suddenly it is later, and you are somewhere else, surrounded by strange faces. Mr. Cohen would in the near future become aware of what had happened and why he was in the hospital, but by then he would be upstairs, there to thank the staff for saving his life. He probably would send them a box of candy.

16

Somewhat bemused, I sat down to write out the man's chart. Although he was feeling well and the immediate crisis had passed, he would require hospitalization. A repeat episode of diving blood sugar might be but a few hours distant.

I picked up the phone to contact the Cohens' physician. The receiver was pressed to my ear and I began dialing. Then the nurse came back, the one who had brought the wife and then returned to flush information from other relatives. She hurriedly grabbed a chair and sat beside me.

"I talked to the family," she said in breathless triumph. "His name is Abraham Cohen, and his wife is Irene. They were arguing about insurance when the old man suddenly passed out. Apparently he just went right down. No warning ... "

"Irene bought Whole Life instead of Term," I replied, listening to the phone ring, "and from a ne'er-do-well cousin. A real nogoodnik."

"What?"

The line was still ringing.

"Do you know about life insurance?" I asked while sliding the incomplete chart before me.

"No, not much," the nurse replied, confused by the change in subject.

"Well, let's just say this," I said, turning to talk to the recently answered phone. "If my wife had done what she did, I would have passed out too ... Hello, Doctor Morris, this is Steve Seager at the Emergency Room. I have a patient of yours, a Mr. Cohen. It seems his blood sugar dipped a little low ..." The nurse said nothing while I was speaking, nor after I hung up. She was still in the same position when I left the room. But she looked at me strangely for the remainder of the evening.

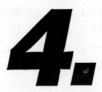

4.

I returned to check Mr. Erickson. His pain had again increased, even in the short time since I had last seen him. Now he was in real agony. His wife, a nicely dressed older woman, held his hand beneath the sheet. Previously, he had been sitting, but now was sunk low in the bed and somewhat curled. This was a bad sign. Regularly, the seated woman would lean over and wipe her husband's brow with an embroidered handkerchief. He was sweating profusely.

His lab results had come back. The white blood cell count was greatly elevated and consistent with his sick appearance. It, and he, indicated that we were dealing with some ongoing infection or injury. I had examined the X-rays, and they were fresh in my mind. One film had shown a loop of large bowel filled with air, a possible indication of some inflammatory process occurring in the area. The loop was in his lower right side. Near the appendix.

I greeted them both. She said hello. He said nothing. I lowered the right-hand bed rail and pulled back Mr. Erickson's sheet. His arm was bent around his stomach; both knees were flexed.

I coaxed him to lie flat. After some doing he managed to straighten out. While gently probing the abdomen I easily found his major source of pain. An area just above the right groin was exquisitely tender, even to a gentle press. He would tolerate no harder thrust. It was the same area that had been abnormal on X-ray and certainly the source of that sky-high white count. If I jiggled his feet or bounced the left flank, his pain was reproduced. The man had appendicitis: I knew that for sure. I also knew that he was spilling pus inside and needed an operation right away.

I have often wished, at times like these, that I had

some vast reservoir of tact from which to draw, or a deep psychological well in which to dip, but I do not. I wish that just the right words, a blend of information and comfort, would somehow spew forth. But they do not. I am by nature blunt and direct, and can only be so. Some people appreciate this approach, others don't. But all get it; it is all I have to offer.

"Mr. Erickson," I began in a tone that immediately made his wife sit a fraction straighter, "you have appendicitis." He didn't budge, or speak. His wife let a small moan escape. I felt awful. No one likes to deliver bad news, even when it is the truth. "And you need an operation."

"Now?" the man said faintly. "Tonight?"

"I'm sorry," I replied, "but, yes, tonight and right now." Before either could react or become lost in emotion I asked some required questions. My queries yielded valuable information and also took their minds away from the immediate shock. "Have you ever been operated upon by any local surgeon? Or do you know someone whom you would like to do the procedure?"

They glanced at one another in silence. The wife turned to me. "Do you have a surgeon here?" she asked.

"Not in the hospital," I said, preparing them for a slight wait, "but we do have one on call. He can be here within the hour if you wish."

"Var?" the nicely dressed woman said, looking toward her husband.

"That will be fine," the ailing man replied, taking control of the situation.

"Good," I uttered smiling, "that will speed things considerably. I'll give him a call."

I finished with a few more questions; no he was not allergic to any drugs, no he had never had a bad reaction to anesthesia, and yes he smoked. This done, I exited. As I swung the curtain closed, I heard both voices talking low.

Back in the station our on-call surgeon was notified. The clerk spoke to his answering service, leaving a message after the correct beep, then hung up. I hoped he would call back quickly. The usual contact time is twenty to thirty minutes. Which càn be a long time if you are in pain.

I sat back to catch my breath. Delivering bad news tires me. Empty charts were staring at me from the rack, evidence of a large number of patients yet to be seen. But they would have to wait, if just for a moment.

My short meditation ended when the ward clerk, our station secretary, angled back in her chair, a phone cradled against one shoulder, and said, nodding to the wedged receiver, "There is a man here who has a cut hand wants to know if it needs stitches."

This is one of our most common phone requests and one for which, of course, there is no answer. Nevertheless we enjoy them every time. The clerk always says the same thing and I always say the same thing. Then we laugh, a good hard laugh. It breaks the tension. We actually look forward to the calls.

"Tell him to hold the cut real close to the phone and have a nurse listen," I said, picking up a handful of charts and walking out.

Prior to any surgery there are certain tests which need to be run. They have over time become routine, like washing one's hands. A blood count and clotting study to determine how much blood the patient has and if it functions correctly. A chest X-ray for a look at the lungs. And a urine and heart check.

Although one spends the time sleeping, surgery is a terrific strain on the body. Thus, prior to beginning, it behooves a surgeon to ascertain precisely what shape his patients are in.

The above-mentioned tests will generally turn up any physical aberration of enough significance to warrant aberration of surgical plans. But, as proved to be the case with Mr. Erickson, sometimes even the discovery of something important will not change the basic decision. It only makes things more difficult.

There are in medicine, as I'm sure in other professions, certain axioms passed like heirlooms from generation to generation—sayings, if you will, given from old physicians to new physicians, terse bits of sage advice accumulated over years of medical practice.

One such homily states, "If you hear hoofbeats, don't look for zebras." This means that common diseases and situations happen most often—that's why they are called common—and should always be suspected first. Everyone knows there are more horses than zebras. The advice is to look for a simple explanation, in any given situation, before launching into an expensive hunt for esoteric pathology. The converse logic applies to rare conditions.

A second maxim is, "Each patient is allowed only one disease." This is, for most intents and purposes, sound advice also. It means that when you are confronted with a puzzling constellation of symptoms, look for a single disease to tie them all together. If you must explain things by invoking two or even three diseases, then chances are you have missed the boat. Look again.

Unfortunately, Mr. Erickson was not privy to these time-honored pearls. For, had he been so, the man no doubt would have exercised the good sense to postpone his heart attack until after his appendicitis.

I spent the lag time between a phone call and surgeon arrival sewing the face of a young teenage man. He was very drunk. I was concerned about Mr. Erickson. This proved to be a bad combination. After much talking and some shoulder pushing the fellow was finally put flat. I had to stitch his torn forehead, a task which required complete cooperation. I did not get it. Repeatedly, after a suture was placed, the inebriated youngster would rise and say, "Are you certain we need to do this?" thereby pulling out the thread. We did this over and over. At first I tried reassurance (yes it was necessary) then humor ("no, but I have a house payment to make and I need the money") finally nothing. I simply forced him down in silence. We were consuming valuable time, and I had many other things to do.

His breath smelled like rancid chicken.

As our needling and sitting progressed, he proceeded, during infrequent lulls, to regale me with details of the evening. While arguing over a twenty-five cent bet, the chap had been struck in the head with a pool cue. Hence the laceration. If he had acted there, as he was acting here, I concluded, I didn't doubt that he deserved to be struck with a pool cue. In fact I was surprised that he had received just one blow. Suddenly, with each sentence he began to grow more heated. As he told again about the actual hit, he became madder and madder. His frustration, unfortunately, was now directed, not at the gentleman who had done the hitting, but at me, the man who was doing the fixing. His language became progressively more foul, his implications more threatening. At last he stated with a sneer, "If this hurts I'm going to punch you in the face."

My temper is long in coming, but hard and fast once reached. He reached it. With a slight tremble I set down my needle holder and grabbed a pair of tissue scissors. Placing one hand squarely on top of the lad's head, I again returned him to the horizontal. I was now perched, albeit upside down, directly above him. I moved in close.

"Do you see these?" I asked, displaying the chrome thread cutters. I felt him nod through my hand. "If you make any move toward me," I said in a voice crackling with emotion, "no matter how small, I mean even a twitch, if you bat your eyelids wrong or make a lip quiver, I will take these scissors and stab them into your eye. Is that perfectly clear?" I added leaning in again. We were now nose to nose. "I mean crystal clear?" I felt another affirmative nod. The rest of the procedure went smoothly.

Why I said that I don't know, even today. I had never been vicious with a patient before. I regret what I did. But even more than that I am eternally grateful that the man chose to lie still, for had he not done so, I surely would have plunged those scissors into his eye. Something snapped inside me, some combination of continuous tension and repressed anger had broken an unconscious barrier. A flood of seething hostility had surged forth. In short, I had lost control.

In retrospect, all I feel is fear. A fear of something buried deep within. Something that sits crouched and waiting to spring. Something I saw that night. Since then, I have practiced piling as much humanity on top of that something as possible, hoping that perhaps a little extra weight will keep the lid on.

5.

As the recently sutured man opened the main door and left, our staff surgeon entered, wearing a tuxedo, cummerbund, and satin pants; he obviously had been at some important social function. Being a friend of his, I knew he hated that type of affair. I knew he would rather operate. And he would get that chance.

"Where is Mr. Erickson?" the surgeon said, undoing his bow tie. It hung like two flat butterflies on his shirt. He reached for and flipped through the chart, stopping briefly to absorb my short note. He also scanned the laboratory reports.

"Steve," he said, handing me the man's cardiogram, "would you look at this while I examine?" I took the folded paper. It was the EKG I had ordered, certain that Mr. Erickson would be going to surgery. It was the EKG that became hoofbeats, the hoofbeats that brought zebras. Lifting my eyes from the page, I let out a low whistle, then looked down the hall. The surgeon was already in with the Ericksons.

When he returned, I knew he was going to wish to be back in the ballroom. "Walt," I said as he picked up the phone and dialed the operating room. There was need to schedule a time and crew and to arrange for anesthesia; he agreed it was a hot appendix. He didn't hear my call, however. "Walt," I repeated.

"Yes, Steve," the dandified man answered.

"Mr. Erickson is having a heart attack," I said in the direct manner that I always use. The same manner that told the Ericksons, among thousands of others, that they needed emergency operations. The same manner I would use again when I told Mr. Erickson about his heart.

With a start the doctor snatched the lined paper from my hand. Holding it at arm's length, he glared long and hard.

He set it on the desk and examined it further. With a pencil I pointed out the salient features, specific areas of cardiac oxygen lack, areas of dying tissue and spots of actual cell death. There was no mistaking the findings. An EKG, like a photograph, rarely lies.

My colleague, the man taken from his dinner, sat down. He placed his chin in both palms. The ante had been upped to house limit. The three of us—an anesthesiologist would make the third—now had to decide which problem to confront first. The choice was tender and agonizing. We were drawing to an inside straight.

Mr. Erickson had two conditions, each potentially fatal. Unfortunately, as is often the case with these situations, the treatment of one ailment almost precluded a successful resolution of the other. It was an awful dilemma. Mr. Erickson not only heard hoofbeats, but the zebras were preparing to trample him.

The surgeon and I talked. If the heart attack were treated with bed rest and observation, as is the recommended therapy, his abscessed appendix would surely rupture, thus propelling infection into every cranny of the man's intestinal cavity. Peritonitis, a severe visceral inflammation, would result. Considering the fellow's age and physical condition, this meant death.

Yet, if the gangrenous bowel tag were removed, the strain of surgery or the effects of sleeping gas might enlarge the heart attack, killing his heart. And him.

The anesthesiologist thanked us for asking him into such a cut-and-dried case. It was, he said, just the thing to fill a dull Saturday night. It was like inviting a straw man to a candle convention, he concluded.

Time, however, was essential to correction of both problems. Either way, a quick decision was required. Briefly the pros and cons for each side were presented. We took a poll. It was decided to operate. If he could somehow survive surgery, we surmised, his chances of living would be far better than if we allowed his appendix to burst and the inevitable peritonitis to develop.

Soon, Mr. Erickson, his tuxedoed surgeon, and the reluctant anesthetist all migrated to the O.R. I did not say good-bye to any of them. There simply was nothing to say. We had decided to operate and the patient consented. I had cast my vote for surgery. It was unanimous.

My attention rapidly turned to other matters, but my thoughts remained upstairs. An ankle sprain was splinted, and a cactus thorn was removed from the seat of a young girl. She had been drinking and sat on the prickly plant.

Then they closed the doors. Not only closed, but locked them as well. This was something that none of us had ever seen done. I watched in amazement as a security guard turned his key from the outside. We were bolted in. I walked to the door and peered out through a small glass pane. The front desk was empty, the waiting room the same. One last woman was being escorted out by a uniformed policeman.

Soon other officers walked through the outside door and carefully made their way down the hall. Their steps were outlined by blips of rotating red light from a police car parked on the ramp. One officer stayed behind and directed newcomers to an area where others were already standing.

I craned my neck another way. Nothing. Everything was empty, except for the police. The place looked like we were closed for the night. A wall clock read 11:45.

"What's going on?" I asked the nearest person, a respiratory technician whom I had seen come in just prior to the door closings. She took me aside with a "shush."

"There is a robbery going on in the pharmacy," the woman said in a low, strained voice, "and they have guns."

"You must be kidding," I replied for lack of anything better.

"No, I'm not," she said.

Our imposed isolation, the locked doors and hushed conversation, ended with the sound of pistol shots.

6.

At times like these I realize that being a doctor, and especially an Emergency Room doctor, is an unusual occupation. This thought first struck me while I was performing a rectal exam. It happened during medical school, a time filled with a good number of unusual experiences.

Medical school is many things. However, like color blindness, it is something only a few people will ever experience and none can adequately explain. In retrospect, it was not a day-by-day happening or a four-year segment of life, but a series of singular and brightly etched pictures, each clear and crisp in detail, yet with no temporal or sequential order. It's like a stack of shuffled photographs or a collection of short stories.

I never reminisce. I'm more content not doing so. But every so often, despite my best intentions, one of these picture stories, full and complete, will flash into my mind and become real once more.

My class was, as a friend said, "like being married to one hundred and fifty people all at the same time." He was right. From my current vantage I can no longer comprehend the sheer volume of time and energy that I expended upon that small group of people. They were an assortment of men and women from around the country, and during those years they were the only persons with whom I had anything to do. They became my sole source of entertainment, amusement, argument, and discussion. In short, my life.

Relationships developed on every level. From the class came friends, enemies, and lovers. Among us were marriages, divorces, fistfights, lawsuits, and suicide. Had we elected a mayor we could have started a town.

The best analogy I can draw is to the movie *Sweet No-*

vember. If you recall, a seriously ill Sandy Dennis takes in, for one month, every month, a new boyfriend. The unsuspecting soul is wined, dined, and romanced. At the end of his month this by now distraught fellow, having fallen in love with her, is summarily dismissed and another fills his place. Such is the case with medical school.

Our term was four years. We, the traveling collection of spouses, were let in, loved, hated, used and abused, taken advantage of and given advantages. We experienced sights and excitements that most people will never know. But, unlike the man in the movie, each of us knew from the start about the deadline, the time when, willing or not, we would be turned out, a new group being directly behind us.

That prospect spawned a general terror. Toward that moment each person inexorably struggled to gather, like plums in a basket, every last bit of fact. We collected knowledge, like so many coins in a sack, as insurance against the day when we would be called "Doctor" and be on our own.

That information was not easily collected. It was extracted only after much sweat and strain, pulled like reluctant onions from huge hard clay medical tomes, heavy sneering volumes which contained, amid multilettered words and multitudinous pages, a storehouse of valuable, well-guarded information. We were taunted by these sophisticated books; learn, or quit.

We fought also, like medieval knights, with vicious examinations, tests administered over time like ancient torture. In preparation, entire nights were spent awake and reading; many meals were spent discussing; many mornings were spent vomiting. For a few, the examinations would demonstrate that, indeed, they were not good enough, that the title of doctor would never be theirs. Those examinations lay blank and smug, like coiled cobras ready to strike. One did not pass or fail them; one conquered them or fled.

In return, as reward to the victors, we got to watch people die. Until a particular September afternoon, I had never seen a dead person, let alone watched one die. My life had been spared the sight of grandfathers passing or uncles collapsing. I had never happened upon a bad car wreck. I had no experience with the dead. The very first day of medical school changed that forever. Since that time I have seen all too many dead persons, and I have seen all too many persons die. I have been witness, not merely to the result, but to the process itself, both quick and long. I have seen death in every conceivable form, even the death of one of our own.

That first day, hot for an Eastern autumn, was filled with anxiety and apprehension. It was like waiting to board an airplane but not knowing where it was going. I realized I was in for an experience yet had no idea of what kind.

The day was marked by two events. One I have noted, and will describe later; I saw a dead person. The second was a crystal-clear appreciation of my total ignorance about the human body.

Medical school is, in its purest form, the study of how the human body works, what can go wrong, and what if anything can be done by way of remedy. I discovered on that first day why this process takes four years.

Lectures began immediately. I barely had time to sit before the room was quiet and the podium filled. The first speaker delivered a talk entitled, "Greetings, and what you should have learned in college." In the course of the rudimentary presentation which followed, mention was made of the adrenal gland. Wishing to clear up a source of mild personal confusion, I turned to a woman seated on my right and asked, "Isn't that the gland in your neck?" She, the apparent recipient of a stronger undergraduate education than mine, remarked with thinly veiled disgust. "No, that is your thyroid. The adrenal gland is on top of your kidney. Your kidney is near your back," she added unnecessarily. I smiled as though I had made a very funny joke. We both knew that I hadn't. I knew I had a long way to go.

When we finally broke for lunch, three lectures later, I noticed the gland woman stop at the door and look back. I have no idea what was going through her mind, and I don't ever care to find out.

After lunch, like frightened cattle, we were led to the Anatomy Lab, where, they said, would be our cadavers. And where, they added, we would dissect them. I looked for the thyroid woman while I fought an uncontrollable urge to say, "Dissection? Isn't that when you cut things up?"

The anatomy professor was a very tall, thin man, much underweight. It is said that eventually dog owners come to look like their pets; in this man's case he had come to look like his job. Except for his pants and shirt, he resembled a used cadaver. Had he lain upon a dissection table, no one would have been the wiser.

I sat far in the back. On purpose. I had arrived early enough to get a closer seat, but after a quick survey of the place I decided I didn't want one. At the front of the room, on a table behind which hung a blackboard, there was a gray vinyl bag. It was the size of a medium-build person. At one end were twin bulges of plastic from which arose other smaller lumps and mounds. My initial assessment proved correct: there was a body in the bag.

I sat as far from the lumpy bag as possible. I wanted a gradual introduction to the dead, nothing too sudden. I was afraid that when the body was removed I would gasp. I had drawn enough attention to myself with that stupid gland comment and was in need of no more.

From the rear, things were not so bad. The unwrapping was ghoulish by any standard to which I was accustomed but not grotesque or painful. The frail, stickbone man unzipped the sack and, like a gardener handling his favorite flower, carefully lifted out the prize.

The body itself was brown like tanned leather but with obvious areas of darkening decomposition. It was a prosection and thus had numerous anatomical structures exposed. It took a while to notice that it was not covered with skin.

My fears about gasping proved unfounded. A gasp, front or back, would have been enveloped by all the rest. When the body emerged everyone gasped. My relief was intense—not only because I had withstood my first encounter with the dead, but because I realized that we all were in the same boat. Even the gland woman. We were all emperors without our clothes, pretending to be something that we were not. We were not doctors, we were children gasping at death. I was even willing to wager that somewhere in that morning lecture a person had turned to his neighbor and asked, "What's a gland?" I felt much better.

There are, I discovered, two types of cadavers. There are new bodies, "virgins," those that have recently died and are as yet uncut. And there are prosections. Prosections are bodies that have been studied by previous classes. Some are used year after year, until they simply wear out, until things are no longer attached to the things which God had intended. Or until things are not in the place that they once were. Or until parts, from repeated handling, simply cease to exist. One cannot learn from a cadaver in this condition; it doesn't correspond to the accompanying manual. When this happens the bodies are replaced with new ones.

The old bodies, the ones studied into submission, are piled onto a cart and burned in the hospital incinerator. One day I happened to see this occurring. Immediately I ran to the window and checked the smokestack. I wanted to know if the smoke had changed color. Medical school, as I said, is an unusual place.

Now I was seeing my first dead body, if only from a distance. That first day's presentation was meant, I suppose, as a foundation upon which to base our further medical studies. As in, "Here is a dead one, now go out and keep the others alive."

The live man filled the afternoon with a lecture about the dead man. He told us how to care for our cadavers. "Keep them wet and well oiled. Use a spoon or brush to paint the body with fat while you are working." He ladled his hand alongside the body as if basting with an invisible spoon. "And be sure to zip the bag when you are done." Dead bodies, like refrigerated sandwiches, will dry unless covered. The professor said other things too. He also wrote on the chalkboard. I know

33

because there was dust in the air. But I was not paying attention. I could not take my eyes off the cadaver.

The learned man had, before starting his dissertation (I'm certain only for convenience), placed the example body, using himself for support, in a sitting position. Every so often as a critical point was reached, he would turn and point out some salient feature on the seated corpse. Midway through, the end of his tie fell into the chest and he never noticed. I guess the fellow was accustomed to having his clothing dangle into dead bodies. I watched the cloth bob up and down, in and out of open ribs, and tried to construct in my mind a conversation between this man and his dry cleaner concerning the spots on his tie. I couldn't do it.

Along with exposed abdominal organs, the dead person's head had been cut in half as well. (One needed to study intracranial anatomy too.) The skull was split lengthwise, cut, I found out later, with a Black and Decker table saw. A clean incision coursed down the forehead, bisecting the nose and making two mouths.

The next instant I will always remember. I have tried over the years to relate it to some larger human equation or draw from it some wise moral conclusion, but I cannot. It just happened.

As the body sat, its head began to waver. Not the entire head, however, but just one side. Then with a swish it dropped. One half of a face fell bouncing onto the chest, the other part remained upright and smiling, as if nothing had happened. If it were possible to describe to you the effect of this, I would. But it isn't.

During our first year we slowly became familiar with the cadavers, a few of whom acquired names, such as Dead Don or Cold Carla, but most of whom just remained cadavers. Initially, some students were less serious than others. One fellow, on a slow Friday, made an intestine lasso and roped his lab partner, but these episodes were few. In general the class was studious and respectful.

As the weeks passed and our hands grew weary, the jokes stopped. Nervous laughter ceased. We began to realize

34

that these bodies were not, as in college, plastic models or rubber replicas. These had once been people, just like ourselves. Only they were dead, and we were not, yet.

From one man's chest we pulled an unexpected surprise, a pacemaker. Someone had worked long and hard at putting that device in. Someone, at one time, cared about keeping that man alive. From another we removed a bullet. Someone, at one time, had wanted this man dead. We found tumors and lumps, broken bones and stumps, all evidence of the human condition, the condition with which these people had dealt and lost, the same condition we were being trained to understand and trained to analyze, the condition we were simultaneously to be above and yet part of.

After our first year we would see no more of the cadavers. On the day we left, they lay, exactly as they had when we arrived, zipped in plastic cases, waiting for the next crop of students, for the next group of young, nervous fingers that would probe, strip, and explore. They waited for the next group of students who would be, as we had been, forced for the first of many times to confront their own fragile mortality.

7.

Suddenly everything was complete confusion. Police-men burst through the once-locked doors and scattered around like ants. The swinging partitions clicked and bobbed with each entering person. Finally they stayed open. Two dangling feet ap-peared, then an officer, moving sideways. He was hefting a bleeding body. Another lawman followed with an identical burden.

Two reclining figures, borne like bags of laundry, were raced down the hallway and thumped into adjoining beds. Both men had been shot. Both were slick with red.

I stood in a nearby cubicle and watched this frenetic procession. I must have been holding a chart because I found one many hours later, kicked into a corner. I looked at the name but could not place the person or remember what we had done for him. I could not recall because the ensuing hours had been so hectic.

I made my way through a clutter of shouting police-men and chattering nurses, at last reaching the central station. Everyone was yelling, and no one could hear anything. Police-men were screaming at the nurses. Nurses were shouting back at policemen. Little was getting done.

"Call the lab please," I asked the unit secretary. "Have them bring tubes for type and cross and H and H." She nodded over the muffling din.

The two H's stand for hemoglobin and hematocrit, tests that measure how many red cells a given blood sample contains and how much hemoglobin (the stuff that transports oxygen) any particular cell carries. Type and cross is a process whereby a person's blood is compared with existing donated samples until an exact copy is found. Precise replication is re-quired before transfusion can begin. And, judging from the twin trails of blood on the floor, transfusion was going to be necessary.

"Excuse me," I said to a group of men in blue. They were squeezed together in the nursing station doorway but parted quickly and let me pass. Before reaching ringside I cut a similar path through other layers of onlookers. Inside this halo of humanity a quartet of nurses, two per patient, were probing the supine bodies with needles. At the head of each bed a respiratory technician was preparing instruments for insertion down the injured men's throats.

I shouted to the head nurse but got no response. A deafening throng of curious spectators, their numbers swelled with pharmacy workers and ambulatory patients had made the scene unmanageable. I was being pressed against a bed rail. An intravenous pole swayed from the jerk of a careless elbow. In desperation I reached across a pair of bloody feet and took a nurse's arm.

"Get these people out of here!" I screamed directly into her face.

"What?" the startled woman called, straining one ear toward me while signaling at the same time in pantomime for another I.V. bottle to be hung.

"GET THESE PEOPLE OUT OF HERE!!" I shouted with words more bark than bellow. My voice was failing. And still the turmoil continued. A second nurse tapped me on the shoulder. I spun around. Through a bird's nest of tangled arms and elbows, I spotted the blood lab technician, the person whom I would need if these men were to receive blood. She was outside the tight circle of gawkers, haplessly pushing against their backs. She couldn't get in.

I wedged down the side of one bed. Finally, near the first man's head, I reached to the top of an intravenous pole and grabbed a bottle, which was dripping salt water into the injured man's arm. The setup was designed to carry blood. Blood carefully matched and typed, to replace what had been spilled on the floor. But the lab woman couldn't get in.

On tiptoes I unhooked the glass container. With a lift it swung free. It was round and firm. It sent a cool tingle through my wet palm. With a burst of angry energy I leaped and flung the fragile receptacle. So hard was my throw that I tumbled forward across an oozing chest.

The resultant shatter was electric. It stole air from everyone's lungs. Sentences were cut. Words drifted out half formed. A silent curtain dropped as tiny bits of glass, swimming in streams of water, tinkled to the floor. A liquid circle, five feet in diameter, appeared on the rear wall.

For a split second I relished the welcome silence, then filled its vacuum with orders. This time, with no contending noise, I didn't need to yell. My audience was wide-eyed and agape. They listened and obeyed.

I cannot recall exactly what I said, but I do remember the crowd backing out like a movie in reverse. In no time the room was clear. There was one more I.V. bottle within my reach. I'm sure that helped.

At last speaking in my normal voice, I asked a nurse to please replace the exploded bottle. Although the container had been destroyed, its plastic tube-line still dangled from the dying man's arm and lay coiled along the floor like a sunburned snake. Ironically, as if sensing my urgent problem, the bottleless tip settled into a pond of the patient's own blood.

Like jack-in-the-boxes, the two respiratory personnel popped up from behind the gurneys, looking at me nervously. Both had gone down when I cocked my bottle-carrying arm. The watermark on the wall was directly behind and between their heads. The aqueous missile had bisected them neatly. Fortunately, each had had sense enough to duck. They went immediately back to work.

With order restored, the lab woman drew both men's blood. Then their venous lines were reattached. Finally, starting with the man in bed one, I began my examinations. The first gentleman had received a bullet in the chest. Each time his mouth opened to breathe, his wound lapped in air like a thirsty dog. I called for the chest tube tray and asked that a bandage be applied. If this man were to live, that blast entrance would require immediate patching, and the air pressure inside would need reequilibration. To do this I inserted a plastic hose through the jagged, yawning puncture and suctioned out his lung cavity.

This chest damage, grave as it was, was but one of the man's problems. Rapid inspection revealed two additional wounds, one penetrating the lower abdomen and the other his right thigh. Each was in itself a major insult. And each needed surgical correction.

With this in mind I ordered another fluid line. Until blood was ready I would replace lost volume with saline, and lots of it. This approach, however, goes only so far. Blood is not only thicker than water but also better. Eventually, without the real thing, my stopgap measures would fail, as would the man.

If things got desperate, as I suspected they might, I had the option of infusing O negative blood. This is transfusion blood that is run in blind, with no laboratory match. It is a special type that carries the smallest probability of causing an adverse reaction. But, even so, allergic sequelae, occasionally fatal, still occur. This would be used only as a last resort.

That choice, however, was eliminated when the blood bank called: the last of this type blood had been used the previous day. Also, the caller added, no source in town was willing to part with its few precious units. Thus I, and my two bleeding companions, had to hope for a regular blood match. Until then, I would continue with water.

Luckily, the treatment of most severely injured patients follows a standard routine. The injuries may vary, as does the manner of their infliction, but their remedies all start with the same things. Everyone needs I.V. fluid, everyone needs laboratory work, and nearly everyone requires breathing assistance. All of this is easily done without one's looking at the patient's face.

A doctor can engross himself in the size of a knife hole or the depth of a gunshot blast. He can gauge the velocity of an attacking truck. He can estimate an amount of blood loss by how large a pool it leaves on the floor. He can read X-rays and phone for consultants. All without looking at a face.

40

Sometimes such avoidance is preferable. There have been times, especially with mutilated children, when I have done just that. But I did not do it then. And I wish I had.

Before moving to the second man, I peered above the first victim's chest. Through a swarth of bandage and between strokes of crimson, I could see the makings of a beard, but a beard in theory only, for it could not have been grown or shaved. I touched his cheek. It was soft, covered with the fine silky hairs of youth. Then I lifted his hands. They too were smooth. Unworked. The hands of someone in school. My head began to pound and my stomach to buzz. Deep cerebral circuits swirled. My feet spun away. This wasn't a man. It was a boy.

There was blood on the floor and water on the wall. And eyes, like those in a bad painting, staring in through the station window. How, I wondered to myself, did a young boy get himself into such a place as this?

Determined to avoid a repeat, I checked the second man in reverse order, beginning with his face. This also proved unfortunate. It made the rest that much worse. After one glimpse my mind went blank, and only slowly stumbled back into gear. From a reserve of instinct I ordered, minus the chest tube, our standard treatment protocol, then proceeded with my evaluation.

In this man's chest, thankfully, I found no holes. Nor any in his arms and legs. He had, it seems, received only one wound, but it was directly to the center of his abdomen. He too would require immediate surgical attention. Finally I stepped away and just looked. The pair lay like wounded warriors, seeping from their battle scars. The boy-man in bed one. And my friend in bed two: our hospital pharmacist.

I looked back into the nurses' station. It was filled to capacity. Policemen were on every phone. Others were animatedly talking to the staff; some were in plain clothing but still appeared to be police. However, the majority of occupants—cop, visitor, and nurse alike—were, like kids before a television set, just watching through the window. Watching the robber the police had shot and the pharmacist the robber had shot. And they were watching me.

8.

In short order the proper surgeons were called. Again we got answering services. Again my nerves jangled as I imagined two doctors either not hearing their beepers or else switching them off in a fit of disgust. The two injured men, the robber and my friend, needed swift attention. I said a silent prayer that the physicians would respond quickly.

That done, I returned to the bedsides. Both patients were still breathing on their own, but doing so poorly. They could continue unassisted for a while, but not for long. I opened the boy's mouth and put in a metal blade. With an upward lift his tongue moved away to reveal an elliptical tracheal orifice. Vocal cords, like fish gills, covered both sides of the passage. I aimed a hollow plastic breathing tube between these tissue vibrators, bypassing the windpipe with no difficulty. I repeated the same steps on the pharmacist. Neither man gagged or vomited. Soon each was receiving full mechanical breaths from hand-pumped bags.

It had been twenty minutes since the shooting and still there was no sign of either surgeon or, as important, of the life-giving blood. I asked the ward clerk to call everyone again. Then I thanked her and began to pace. I paced while intravenous lines dripped in a race against the clock and doctors' beepers. As I watched blood well from metal-shredded arteries onto our patterned vinyl floor, it appeared as if that race was going to be lost.

When the phone calls finally came, it was just like the "good news–bad news" jokes. I always ask for the good news first, and that is what the ward clerk gave me. The good news, she said, was that one surgeon had called back and was on his way. "What's the bad news?" I replied. She said nothing but pointed to a blinking light on the telephone. I nodded and picked up the receiver. It was the blood bank. And it was bad news.

People think of their blood as one of a few alphabetical types and, in general, this is true. They are familiar with the ABO system and know that a "positive" or "negative" is added. As in, "I have 'A positive' or 'B negative' blood." There are, however, other matching systems, which are equally important for transfusion matching. When one considers these additional systems, the chances of two random persons having an exactly identical blood type are remote. But not impossible, as I found out.

Both of my bleeding men had the same blood type. Not just for ABO, but for everything, exactly, right down the line. And it was rare. Just four units could be located, barely enough, barring complications, to squeak one patient through a major operation. "Perhaps," I asked, "another source could be found? Another hospital? Or blood bank maybe?" The woman agreed to try but, considering the time element involved, she said finding any extra seemed unlikely.

I sat on a stool and rubbed my forehead. It was oiled and shiny. A thin sheet of sweat greased my fingers. I was perspiring from the heat of overhead lights and the weight of decision. I had surgeon and blood enough for one. But which one?

The surrounding conversation swirled into an indistinguishable buzz, like the sound of a thousand angry bees. Millions of air molecules pounded on my eardrums. My temples burned. The two violated bodies smeared into a myopic blur. I thought back to last summer, when I would often float in my pool, staring into the sky, wondering which cloud might duck behind the porch eave first.

Even after the precious blood arrived, all four units, I still just sat. A nurse, red packs in hand, asked where she should hang one. I told her to set up, but not connect. She went to the bedsides and began work. I was stalling and we both knew it. A decision was needed, and fast. It was needed before the surgeon arrived. To wait for him would be passing the buck. And what if we disagreed? I was determined to choose, start the blood, and present one savable patient to the cutting doctor.

I have always been irritated by people who say that doctors "play God." I have no conception of what that means. A physician is presented with situations in which a decision is required. Many times the problems are complex and the results of immense importance. Often moral, ethical, and even legal dilemmas arise, and they are all considered. But in the end a decision must be made, and someone has to make it.

Is this "playing God"? Is choosing who will live and who will die "playing God," when a choice has to be made? Perhaps. Perhaps not. But that night, had I not chosen, both men would have died.

I cannot recall my exact reasoning process or if there even was one. Maybe I flipped a mental coin. Or drew between a long and a short cerebral straw. I don't remember. I do, however, remember the nurse standing between both men with the blood transfusion ready, the tubing poised, staring in through the glass and waiting.

I looked at the boy in bed one. He was no more than sixteen. He had on blood-stained tennis shoes, nearly treadless on the bottom. I imagined the hours of basketball that had thinned those rubber soles. But tonight he had worn them to steal drugs. There were needle marks on his arms.

The man in bed two had worked at the hospital for as long as I could remember. I had spoken to him often as he stocked our shelves. We always discussed movies or chatted about sports. I had seen his face many times before. How I wished that I had not seen it tonight.

I would like to say that my eventual choice was based on cold hard reason. That I carefully weighed the boy's future against the man's family and arrived at the best conclusion. I would like to think that emotion played no part. But this was not the case. I nodded toward bed two. My friend the pharmacist would receive the blood and immediate surgical attention. He would be given the chance to live. The boy in bed one, the stranger, was on his own. He would have to survive on intravenous water until it would sustain him no longer. Then, barring an unlikely miracle, he would die.

One of the ironies of Emergency Room work is its utter disregard for timing and sensibilities. Often the most cruel and bitter situation will be followed by the funniest. You come to realize that things are, after all, relative. Somewhere someone is always dying and somewhere someone is always laughing. How your life goes is merely the frequency with which you happen to be in, one spot or the other.

As I sat watching the pharmacist live and the thief die, I heard three loud, shrill screams. I didn't move but simply laid my head down. I had had enough. I honestly did not want to know what was going on. But, as is always the case, like it or not, I found out. The head nurse, an aide, and two policemen ran to see what had happened.

The group was gone for five minutes. They returned laughing, not giggling or chuckling, but roaring. They were convulsing away the enormous tension that had built up over the blood decision. Although everyone had not participated in its making, everyone shared in its agony. A release was needed. And that release unwittingly found its way to the front door.

The screeches had come from our now beleaguered receptionist. She had seen a man run up the auto ramp and stop, then look around as if confused. Perhaps he was searching for a door handle, she thought. Then he stepped onto the electric eye pad and both glass panes slid open. Instead of entering, however, he remained standing in the doorway. The pair were now face to face, not twenty feet apart. With a flurry, the gentleman opened his coat. He was naked. The receptionist screamed.

Having received what he had come for, the fellow calmly buttoned his jacket and fled. The startled woman continued to scream. Then to laugh. And laugh. Finally, she was laughing so hard that she could barely relate the details of her experience. With each sentence a new wave of mirth washed through her speech, scrambling the words. Soon the others were laughing also, as laughter infects those who listen despite having no idea why they are laughing.

At last her story was complete. Everyone at the desk wiped tears from their eyes. One of the policemen caught his breath long enough to ask the color of the flasher's hair. He was trying to gather information for a report. "Brown," the weary woman answered, twirling in her swivel chair. "He had brown hair."

"And what did he look like?" the lawman continued in some semblance of a normal voice. The woman stopped and pondered before answering. "I don't know," she replied, "I didn't see his face." Again everyone erupted into laughter, louder, if that were possible, than even the first time.

9.

Medicine, in a nutshell, is a series of decisions. Some easy, some hard. The blood decision had been hard. Learning to make it was even more difficult.

Despite the Emergency Room's noise and commotion, you as a doctor are alone. As when walking on a crowded street in a strange city, you can be surrounded by people but you are still alone. There are others with whom you may talk. Or laugh. Or cry. But there is no one else to help you make a decision. There is just you. Other eyes turn and see you. You turn and see nothing.

To survive all alone you must learn three things: how to choose, how to act, and how to stand. For some new doctors each of these steps occurs singly and over a long period of time. For others they come all at once. A few always knew. A few never will.

For those unfortunates who must wait for this knowledge, it can be a very difficult time indeed, a time in which self-confidence can erode to stubble. A number of people in my intern class considered quitting mid-way through. They simply could not bear the weight of standing alone.

As much as possible, I have come to know myself, my capabilities and liabilities, where I am comfortable and where I am not. I have, I believe, accumulated the three attributes. But in the beginning this was not so.

Throughout medical school I saw scores of patients. Since then I have seen an equal number. But there is a big difference between the two groups. They are as separate as opposite lanes on the freeway. In school, no matter what the problem, there was always another physician, an experienced resident or seasoned staff man with whom I could consult, someone to whom I could sound off my ideas, a person to whom I could pass my burden with a relieved sigh. In short, when I turned, someone was there.

This idyllic, womblike cocoon continued until the final day, right up through caps and gowns. Then things were different. Graduation, which had seemed so far away, finally arrived. When it came, the supporting doctors were gone, and I was on the other side of the road. Glancing around I saw oncoming headlights. They had left me alone.

Medical school graduation was an exultant, effusive experience, a day of unbridled self-indulgence and pride. It was an ecstatic calm before the storm. It was to be my last free moment. A tornado of doubt waited outside to blow me away.

The sun that day was a brilliant, burning diamond embedded in a ring of blue sky. The air was light and soft. It was like no other day before or since. I walked from the school building, where a parent-student reception had been held, to the Symphony Hall, where the proceedings were to take place. My flowing black gown and matching hand-held hat reflected the warm afternoon light. They were a symbol to the world, a sign that I had met the challenge and made the mark, that I had bitten off what the academic world had to offer and chewed it to everyone's satisfaction. I was about to step onto the top of the pile. And I loved it. I was about to become a doctor.

The actual ceremony was rich in regalia and ceremony. A flood of proud relatives popped flash bulbs at our broad smiling faces. Wagnerian tunes were played. A visiting dignitary delivered an address. We were seated behind him and didn't hear a word. Then, one by one, we filed to the front as our names were read. From a somber man, each of us received a piece of rolled paper. A rousing march began and we left in unison, the flash poppers following.

The front sidewalk immediately swarmed with black, tipping hats and flapping capes. Parents clustered about like moths and took more pictures. In time the bunch began to scatter. With each departing cluster our knot of enthusiasts became smaller, until, with a final carload, all were gone. The street, at last, was empty.

There would be times in the future, especially that first night alone, when I would long to be back on that street. To shake again those congratulating hands and reflect those Kodak bursts. To turn my face to the sky and stand frozen. Forever.

I was fortunate; I learned my very first day in the other lane. For me all the agony and self-doubt were expended during one single night, my first as a doctor, and on one single patient, also my first as a doctor.

I arrived to start my internship white-coated and smiling. I was a doctor but in name only. I hadn't yet passed through the gauntlet of emotion, that trial by fire, which comes to every physician. That moment when you stand alone, and either sink or swim.

My moment came that first night. And I swam.

It is difficult to describe the feeling of being a new doctor, of knowing that you are the only one to care for all those people—the people who up until then had been just numbered charts, interesting diseases, or bodies upon which to press while a wiser man lectured. Suddenly these people were patients. And patients on whom I would have to press in earnest, without the benefit of lecture.

It is, I suppose, like sailing a hang glider that you have built by hand, over which you have strained for many years, one which no one, yourself included, is certain will fly. There is a certain feeling in your chest as your feet leave the ground, and you look down.

I drew night-call that first day and by 6:00 P.M. everyone had gone. All the old and new doctors. The old were tired, the new were relieved. Relieved that it was me and not them being left behind.

Each one, before he abandoned ship, had given me a report on his patients, a list of what sick people were where, what was wrong with each of them now, and what might go wrong with them later. Then they left.

I tried eating dinner, but the cafeteria food stuck in my mouth like old library paste. Somehow one disagreeable lump found its way to my stomach before I returned a full tray to the kitchen.

As I headed back to the floor my beeper sounded. With it my heart jumped. My back instantly ran with water. I began to breathe hard and feel faint. I leaned against a wall, and mercifully the episode passed. But the beeper continued. I was needed in the Intensive Care Unit.

A local man had become ill while visiting relatives away from home. Refusing reasonable advice to seek medical help there, he started back, with his wife. She drove; he lay in back. When they started, they were 120 miles away from us.

As they traveled, a sharp pain in his chest worsened, his breathing became more shallow and labored. The windows were rolled down. Twice the pair pulled over. For unknown reasons this seemed to precipitate some improvement. They passed two other hospitals on the way. At last the car pulled up to our door. She was hot and exhausted. He was blue and gurgling. He was the man I was called to see.

At that particular hospital there was no actual Emergency Room. A Medical Officer sat in a small cordoned-off area near the main door. Every night one of the full-time staff physicians manned this lonely post. That night there was a psychiatrist on duty.

After seeing the gasping man in the backseat, the only person more nervous than myself was the psychiatrist. He looked in the newly arrived car, closed the door, and ordered everyone upstairs. Perhaps, a nurse suggested, it would be easier if they removed the man from the car first. I think the flustered doctor wanted them to drive to the Intensive Care Unit. Fortunately, cooler heads prevailed. The patient was placed on a cart and wheeled into an elevator.

In the unit, the man was hastily lifted into a bed. From a distance I could see that he was in bad trouble. I could also see the psychiatrist peering in from the hall. He was sweating more than the patient. I hustled to the bedside.

Even for a neophyte it did not take long to ascertain that this fellow had an unusual condition. It looked like something about which I had read but never seen. Something, I learned later, that some physicians never see. As nearly as I could tell, fluid had accumulated around his heart. He had a problem called "cardiac tamponade." A fancy name for liquid accumulating inside the heart's saclike pericardial covering, a name for a lot of water in a small space. And a name for death if it was not soon drained.

If I could assume my diagnosis to be correct, relief of this water tension would solve the problem. Were I wrong, however, the siphoning procedure, a needle pushed through the chest, could induce any number of severe complications, each, given his current state of health, leading to possible death.

It was at this moment that I questioned my decision to become a physician. And thought about the graduation sidewalk.

I reexamined the man's chest and reread his electrocardiogram. I looked again at his chest X-ray. I was only postponing the inevitable. I was hoping that if I searched hard enough or waited long enough, something would change. I was hoping that somehow his symptoms would evolve into a more familiar syndrome or an easily treatable disease. I wished for a sickness I had seen before.

After a second check, and a quick third, my answer was still the same. In fact, the diagnosis only became firmer. I knew there was fluid in his chest, strangling his heart.

From this ailing man I learned to trust my judgment. To consider the options, reflect, and act. From this man I also learned a lesson about life and death, and the fickle unexplainable nature of both. I learned that things are not always as they seem.

Summoning an uncertain courage, I asked the nurse for a long needle and a syringe large enough to hold the fluid I trusted was in my patient's chest. The assembled apparatus was handed to me. I tested the plunger. It slid easily. Placing the lance tip just below the man's rib cage I stopped for a breath. The microscopic hairs on my neck were standing, the large tendons behind my knees contracting. I placed one foot on the bed and pushed the needle in, advancing a steel spike through another person's body.

The metal disappeared up and under his ribs until it was completely gone. For an instant there was nothing. Sweat sprouted on my back. The assisting nurse unconsciously bit her lower lip. Then, with a rush, the suction broke. The syringe surged with straw-colored fluid. Just as I had planned. In a matter of minutes the hidden, heart-killing water was harmlessly swirling in a basin. The man took three long breaths, sat up, and spoke in a calm voice. He waved to his wife. He smiled.

But for the support of the bed under my leg, I would have collapsed. As it was, my heart was racing and my eyes were blurry. I excused myself and went into the hall to sit down.

The near-deadly fluid was sent to the lab for routine examination, a standard procedure. Regrettably, the result was not so standard. When a pathologist looked at the effluence under his microscope, he found a multitude of cancer cells. It was fatal fluid after all.

We took another chest X-ray. In an area originally obscured by the swollen bag of fluid there was a lung tumor. Plans were made to operate but we never got the chance. The man I'd saved once died too soon.

Exactly one week to the hour after I rescued him, I pronounced him dead. Again it was night and again I was alone. As I pulled the sheet over his morbid clay face, I thought of all my labored reasoning and dreadful emotion. I thought of the smooth, sleek slide of that shining needle through the sick man's chest. I remembered my relief and boyish thrill at finding fluid.

And for what? To save a man so he could die of cancer? I had stopped a quick, unannounced death and delivered instead an agonizing, expected torture. I had taken him off the express and put him on a slow, painful train.

A malignant lung cancer had invaded the man's heart,

54

causing fluid to be secreted, fluid that should have killed him but didn't, because I saved him—so that cancer could kill him.

It took a while, perhaps the better part of a month, to sort things through. I spent many hours in a quiet room rubbing one palm against the other and staring. I thought again about the years and the lectures, the patients and the problems. I remembered that sunny sidewalk and my cap and gown.

Then it hit me. Finally I understood about fluid and cancer and the pomp of graduation. I knew they had been my steps toward obtaining the three attributes: how to choose, how to act, how to stand. Never again would there be another time like that. Never again would I look inside myself and wonder. I would always be alone. But it didn't matter.

10.

The first surgeon arrived and examined his patient. He glanced over at the other man but asked no questions. For that I was grateful. With machinelike precision an operating room was scheduled and made ready. Then the doctor was off to scrub. Soon the pharmacist, with breathing machine pumping and blood tube dripping, was gone also. Gone to have his abdomen opened. Gone to get his bleeding stopped.

No sooner was my friend away than the overhead speaker system sounded. The thick gravy air was broken by an electronic snap. It was the paging operator engaging her microphone. The sound caught your attention like a dance announcer when he blows into a mike to see if it's on. Everyone turned toward the crack. There were no routine announcements this late. Only emergency broadcasts were heard at night.

The original snap was followed by a high nucleonic squeal. People sucked in air. Then came urgent words, loud and shrill, in cutting contrast to the vespertine stillness. The deliverer's voice had that nasal twang so common to persons who speak over amplified systems. She had the tone and inflection that made the number "nine" into "niyen." "Code arrest in Surgery ... Code arrest in Surgery," the operator said in her anonymous metallic voice. This was followed by two ringing bells, much like a cheap doorbell, then the message was repeated.

Quickly the E.R. staff was in motion. In a learned response, the appropriate people grabbed the appropriate instruments and ran. They were out of the department and on their way by the time the doorbells were sounding. The second spoken message fell upon few ears. Only some straggling visitors and a slowly sweeping janitor looked up at the ceiling as if seeing the actual speaker box would somehow make things clearer.

I was one of the people hustling to surgery, walking briskly, having learned long ago not to run. During medical school the younger residents and interns used to run, but that stopped when one of them fell and broke his leg. Besides, if there is any distance to cover, and especially if stairs are involved, it takes two or three minutes of bent-over panting after you get there before you can be of any help. It is best simply to walk apace with your eyes peeled for obstacles.

A security guard was holding an elevator for all the emergency personnel. I was last on the car. "Surgery, please," I said upon entering. Everyone laughed. This is a small joke I play everytime there is a code arrest and a car full of people waiting to get there. It always gets a chuckle and relieves a good deal of nervous tension.

In the hospital when someone's heart stops beating or his breathing ceases, an emergency team is rapidly summoned. This scenario, for reasons entirely unknown to me, is called a "code arrest." The arrest part I understand: a nonfunctioning heart is said to be "in arrest." It is the word "code" that is unclear. I would imagine this to be a unique twist of meaning, common only to the medical world. The situation has been further complicated by shortening the description to simply, "a code," leaving out the arrest part entirely. And there is more. When a patient's vital functions cease, he is not dying, he is "coding." "Call a code!" someone will shout while pumping on a failing person's chest. This is not, however, the same as "calling a code"; "calling a code" means stopping a code already in progress, that is, calling it off. An entire idiomatic construct has developed, with an array of jargon expressions and peculiar syntax, all aimed at avoiding the word "death."

Once upstairs, we new arrivals were hastily thrown into surgical gowns and had gloves thrust upon our hands. Masks were strapped at odd angles over our faces. We were given paper shoe covers. All of this was a superficial gesture toward maintaining a sterile atmosphere. We all knew this was more routine than necessary. If the patient survived long enough to get an infection he would be extremely lucky.

I was taken by surprise when I saw the patient. It

58

was Mr. Erickson. For some reason I was shocked. It wasn't that I had forgotten him, it just seemed like such a great while since he had left. Hadn't it been yesterday? Or last week? A quick glance at the wall clock told me that other things really hadn't taken all that long. The shooting episode and its blood decision had been so intense, that they had swelled with time,like a sponge, expanding to destroy any real sense of minute or hour.

Now I was swept with competing emotions. The dying man was Mr. Erickson, a situation, considering his condition, not entirely unexpected; it was not the pharmacist. On the elevator I had prayed that it would not be my friend. That would have made things unbearably difficult. For had it been the pharmacist coding, my blood decision would have been incorrect. The two units already run would have been wasted, and both men condemned to die. But it wasn't the pharmacist, it was Mr. Erickson. I guess my prayer was answered.

In a moment it all came back to me, the tender abdomen, the curled knees, and the well-dressed woman. I don't like to think that I was glad Mr. Erickson was dying, but I must admit, the pharmacist would have been worse. As a team we went to work.

An operating room nurse was already pumping the man's chest, forcing blood from his inert heart by pressing with extended arms and flat palms, like a piston. The anesthesiologist was operating an in-place breathing tube. He was also calling medication orders to a second nurse. Every so often this other nurse would push a prepackaged ampule of clear liquid into Mr. Erickson's intranvenous line. Then everyone except the chest presser would step back and stare at an overhead cardiac monitor. When no change was evident they would reassemble around the bed until another call for medicine was given.

The surgeon was not involved in the resuscitation effort. He was hastily suturing the final inches of an abdominal incision. Stitches were falling amid a churning stomach sea caused by the repetitive thorax compressions. His knots were loose and large, needle holes uneven. With each new thrust, he cursed—and for good reason. Mr. Erickson had nearly made it through the operation. He had, in fact, actually survived the surgery part; his heart gave out while he was being closed up. The surgeon had managed to guide this man through an hour and a half of controlled trauma, but doctor and patient were tripped at the finish line.

I offered advice as it seemed appropriate, and twice administered medication directly into the dying man's heart. Those with me took turns pushing the chest and drawing up drugs.

"Calling" some codes is easier than others. Halting efforts on a decrepit nursing home resident or a person with terminal cancer is easy. With young people, or those to whom you have developed emotional ties, it is difficult. A tiny voice inside says, "Just one more medicine" or "Two more minutes." Perhaps, you think, another procedure will turn the corner. All doctors have seen cases in which a patient has been coded for long periods of time and somehow survives. They could not have done this, the little voice says, if the code had been stopped. So things go on.

Eventually, long after life, the voice stops. Suddenly, pumping on a broken chest and forcing air into a blue face seems ludicrous. An uneasy look passes among the group. The fight for life has gone on too long. There are comments made about the dignity of dying and about the futility of it all. Still, we all know that next time things will be precisely the same. I guess it is human nature.

Unfortunately, that is what happened this night. A multitude of medicines were given but to no avail. The strain of surgery had finally become too much for Mr. Erickson's newly damaged heart. The organ had given out and would not be revived.

"That's enough, don't you think?" I said. The surgeon and anesthetist agreed. Then, like mourners at a funeral, we walked single file out the door. For a while no one spoke. The surgeon jerked off his rubber gloves and flipped them angrily across the hall. They hit the opposite wall with a thud and dropped to the floor.

We walked slowly back downstairs. Gowns and gloves were peeled off. I pulled my mask down around my neck. Cool air bathed my sweat-damp face. Talk was of sports and the weather, not about Mr. Erickson. I contributed little. I was trying to compose my words for the dead man's wife.

As the waiting room got closer, I began to walk rigidly and take smaller steps. Everyone had trickled away save one nurse and myself. We would go in together. Since I had known the woman best (meaning I had spoken to her twice), I was selected as spokesman. "Besides," the nurse added seriously, "you've had the most practice."

We hesitated in the doorway, then entered. Mrs. Erickson's head was lowered, looking at a magazine but she quickly jerked it up. Her eyes were round and filled with premonitory dread. She knew what I was going to say. A lump the size of a tennis ball grew in my throat. It raised the pitch of my voice. I forgot what I had rehearsed and said simply, "Mrs. Erickson, the operation did not go well. Your husband is dead." I followed this with a few words of minor consolation and told her that I would be back to answer any questions she might have. "The nurse will help you choose a mortuary and get anything that you need," I concluded, then excused myself, vowing to apologize later to the nurse for leaving so swiftly.

I could hear the anguished woman's sobs far down the hall. They did not blend into the cradling airconditioner hum and become indistinct until I was well behind the closed swinging doors and near the rear of the Emergency Room.

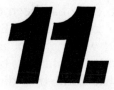

11.

The department was once again full. Seven of eight beds were occupied and everyone was waiting for me. The chart rack was overflowing with clipboards, all of which had blank paper attached. At the top of each paper was a person's name and a one-line summary of his complaint. I picked up the first one. It said "Bitten by monkey." I missed the name. My forehead wrinkled and I looked at the clock. It was 3:30 A.M. A nurse shrugged her shoulders. I looked out the station window. A young man in bed three had his hand pressed against the side of his neck. His shirt was torn into two large segments with many smaller tatters and frays. I noticed a policeman in the same cubicle.

Quickly I thumbed through the remaining charts, looking for anything that seemed serious. The head nurse pointed out a man in bed one who was just being hooked to the heart monitor. There was an ambulance cart beside him, as well as the vehicle's two attendants. One was folding a sheet and generally cleaning up, the other was holding a paper for the ailing man to sign. He was also requesting payment for the ride. I knew this was occurring because I heard the ambulance man mention Master Charge. This kind of thing happens all the time. Many people call an ambulance in the panic of a crisis which, until it is resolved, makes them forget about money. I know that if the company does not make a profit there will be no ambulances to call. Still, sometimes they go too far. This was one of those sometimes. I had a nurse shoo the drivers away and asked our clerk to order an EKG.

Then I asked about the young robber. His bed was empty and since I had not seen him in the hall, we must have passed in opposite elevators, he going up and I going down.

I knew he hadn't died because no code had been called. One of the nurses said that while I was away with Mr. Erickson the second surgeon had been spotted walking through the main lobby. He had been in the neighborhood when his beeper went off. Instead of stopping to call he had come over directly.

Although none too pleased with the circumstances, such as the lack of blood, the doctor had nevertheless agreed to attempt a curative procedure. An operating room was engaged, ironically, the same suite just vacated by Mr. Erickson.

At my request, the unit secretary phoned upstairs to check on their progress. The boy was already on the table, the clerk said, and being prepped for incision. Quietly I wished him good luck and went to see the monkey bite.

Once in cubicle three I saw why a policeman was present. The patient was handcuffed to the bedrail, his left arm draped over the metal rod to which the cuffs were attached, his right hand held against his neck.

"Hello," I said, pulling the curtain around. I got no reply.

"What happened?" I asked, again practicing my vow to keep a straight face during these situations. Still the man said nothing. I looked to the officer for help.

"Mr. Hancock here," the policeman said, tipping the end of a pencil toward the silent man, "held up a convenience store tonight." The lawman was completing some sort of form and looked up only infrequently as he spoke. There was, however, a grin on his face all the while. "And, although he successfully eluded a police chase, the suspect was apprehended by a monkey on Dexter Avenue. And I must admit," the lawman said, lowering his writing implement, "the monkey did a very nice job, a very nice job indeed." He smiled benevolently at the chagrined robber.

The cop was playing his scene for all it was worth. This was obviously the most enjoyable thing that had happened to him all night and, I had to admit, once I heard the entire story, it did wonders for me too.

The handcuffed man had robbed an all-night market. After loitering around the greeting card rack and grazing among the candy bars, he made his move. When the last week-end beer buyer had departed, the man approached the counter. Setting down a can of soda and a Mars bar, the young fellow reached back as if to find his wallet. Instead he produced a knife.

The clerk, a girl no more than twenty, stopped ringing the register and let out a scream, then knocked over a stack of *TV Guides.* She was quickly shushed by the holdup man, who rearranged the magazines. The bandit demanded that the till be emptied. This was done—yielding all of thirteen dollars and eighty five cents—while he vaulted the counter and filled a grocery bag with liquor. Nothing more was said between the two. In approximately three minutes the man was gone. He had, however, neglected to see the girl press a silent alarm with her foot. As the thief rounded the building and dashed across an open field, the police were already pulling into the parking lot, spraying tiny bits of gravel against the front window.

The investigating officer, the man I met in the Emergency Room, said that he was impressed with how calmly the young checker had handled this distressing event. She did not seem the least bit flustered, but gave an accurate description of the culprit and pointed out the direction in which he had fled. All the while she was eating the bandit's Mars bar.

Quickly two officers were off in hot pursuit. Halfway across a weed-infested plat they found the bag of liquor bottles. One was broken, having smashed against a hidden rock. The man had dropped any extra weight once he knew a chase was imminent. While examining the bag, the pursuers spotted their quarry ducking into an alley between two nearby buildings. Scraping sagebrush from their pants, the hunters were soon at the alley entrance. Then they stopped. The alcove was extremely long and, as far as either could see, bordered on both sides by high block-fencing. The suspect had obviously scaled one of the adjoining walls and taken off in a tangential direction. It appeared the hunt was at an end. It would have been impossible to lumber over each barrier and search every yard. Besides there was no moon out and the lighting was poor.

The two men stood for a moment, then prepared to return to their car. That's when they heard the screams. The night air was suddenly filled with a man's terrified pleadings and an infernal howl. This cacophony was interspersed with the clank of rolling garbage cans and the crash of falling debris. Both officers ran toward the noise.

At the site of commotion, the fence changed from stone to wire, affording the constables a clear view into the yard.

They arrived just in time to see the holdup man hurl another refuse can from his perch on a barbeque grill. The container thumped to the ground and spun on a cement patio. As it turned, wet garbage plopped out. The twirling bin crashed into two previously thrown cans behind which was the object of this bombardment, a very excited monkey. Not, the policeman said, a small monkey but a large muscular one, probably a chimpanzee. The animal, as big as a large child, seemed capable of inflicting a good deal of harm upon someone, and it appeared he had chosen to do just that to the robber.

The attacking chimp leapt over the trash cans and made one final advance. He was repelled by flying charcoal briquets. Both officers were too amused to notice anything else. They did not hear the other monkeys chattering from inside a nearby cage nor did they see a flashlight appear.

A fourth man emerged from the rear of the yard. He unlocked an intervening gate, all the while directing the light upon the wrathful monkey. This diverted the animal's attention from the barbecue stand. By the time the creature was collared, both policemen were over the fence and identifying themselves. The thief was down from his precarious perch and voluntarily standing between the men in blue.

In short order the situation was explained. The owner put his monkey back in a cage. The chimp, he said while locking an iron door, occasionally got out, especially when lockup was left to his wife, as it had been that night. The man said that he ran a menagerie and that there were other, more docile, animals kept in the next yard. He shined his light through a side fence and illuminated a collection of covered cages.

The officers apologized for the inconvenience. The animal man invited the policemen to bring their children for a free visit. The robber asked if they couldn't please leave.

Now I lifted the man's hand and saw a nasty neck laceration underneath. It ran nearly the entire length of his jaw and curled down to include part of his chin. It would require a plastic surgeon, I stated. Still the thief said nothing. I explained to the officer exactly what would transpire and approximately how much time would be consumed.

As I walked back to the nurses' station, I couldn't help but chuckle. I thought of the surprise this fellow must have experienced when he leaped over a dark fence and into the arms of that monkey. Then I laughed out loud.

The man with chest pain, the one badgered about his bill, was having a heart attack. The EKG done while I was hearing the monkey story showed unmistakable evidence of heart muscle damage. There was also an occasional extra beat. He was given medication to quiet the unwanted contractions and rolled away to the Coronary Care Unit.

Fortunately the remaining cases required little time to complete. An assortment of colds, a sore throat, and a headache that "just wouldn't quit" were seen, treated, and sent home. Then, for a brief moment, all was quiet. In a distant corner a plastic surgeon was suturing the monkey victim's face. An overhead light concentrated its beam into a spotlight on his hands. Like a youngster at a ball game, the policeman sat quietly and watched. Occasionally there were bits of conversation exchanged among the three.

But still no word from surgery.

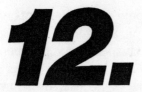

12.

When I first began emergency work I was amazed at the number of intoxicated patients. On a weekend that figure might approach fifty percent. A lot of the people have been in fights, others in accidents, major and minor. Most are cut, bruised, or broken. And they are all mad. Mad at themselves, mad at an assailant, mad at their car, or just mad in general. Regardless of the situation, I patch my drunken friends and turn them out to drink again, to fight again, and, unfortunately, to drive again.

I don't drink. Whenever I am at a party or visiting someone's home I am invariably offered alcohol; I refuse it, and then feel compelled to give some excuse for doing so. Almost without exception that reason is weak and far from the point. It is not very often that I can describe my feelings about alcohol or explain the truth. Rarely will I tell anyone that I don't drink because I hate alcohol. I hate it because of what it makes me see. Quietly taking a soda is so much simpler.

The respite provided by the monkey man proved short-lived. I did not even have time to phone upstairs before Michael B. arrived.

I don't know all that much about Michael B. really. I was with him such a short time and soon there were others who needed my attention. I do know, however, that he owned a blue car, because that is what the paramedic said. I also know that Michael B. was wearing a gray suit with a matching striped tie.

He had been carrying a wallet. It lay on the counter next to his chart. The leather was cracked and worn flat. Inside the billfold were credit cards, some creased receipts with faded numbers, and a stack of folded pictures.

The pictures were in that special compartment all wallets have, the one where people also keep their driver's license. The police had removed Michael's license, but they left the pouchful of pictures.

The photos were of two small children, a girl and, I believe, a boy—with the little one it was hard to tell. There was one snapshot of an attractive woman. She was Michael's wife. I know that because I met her later the same night.

Michael B. was nearly home when he noticed a friend's car parked at an after hours tavern. He looked sober enough when he first arrived, the bartender said, but proceeded to drink heavily over the next two hours. He "seemed all right" when he left, the man behind the counter told police.

No one saw Michael get into his car. It was not until a passing motorist watched him skid off the road that he was found again. A woman said that she saw the car swerve slightly but that it did not appear to be out of control. The automobile came to rest on the gravel shoulder. The man who eventually got out looked drunk, she continued. The police thanked the lady for her time and attention to detail.

Of all the people involved, the truck driver was most shaken and thus remembered the least. As the two officers talked at the hospital, I heard them mention him only briefly. One said that he felt sorry for the fellow. The other agreed.

To some, I imagine, drunken people are amusing, what with lampshades on their heads and all. Granted, drinking does soothe jangled nerves. It is different things to different people. But still very few persons grow to hate it. I think this is because so few people see, or are willing to talk about, the alcohol story's conclusion. For most people the alcohol tale is like a movie that you leave in the middle: you laugh a little, cry a little, figure out the plot, hate the villain, but miss the punch line. Very few people get the full effect. Very few people stay around for the end. I do, a lot. And Michael B. did.

Before leaving the bar, Michael B. telephoned his wife to say that he was on his way. She begged him to be careful and said that she loved him. It was not until thirty minutes later, when her husband still had not arrived, that she became worried. As if by fate the woman called our hospital first.

I wonder if he thought about his children as he was asking for another round or careening down the road. They were very cute, just like their pictures. The boy was now recognizable as a boy, having grown some since the wallet photo. He wore pajamas with long sleeves and feet. "Mork from Ork" was written on the shirt. Even this late the lad was smiling.

The girl, older than her brother, sensed that something was wrong. She peered nervously from behind her mother's legs. She looked like a porcelain doll in her pink satin robe.

I saw the children again while they were sitting in a side room. At first, neither of them noticed me as I stopped to watch. The boy, age two (I know because my son is that age), was beating the floor with a rolled magazine and singing. He wasn't singing a real song, but just making sounds, the kind of sounds that children make when they are preoccupied or bored. The girl was sitting on the couch. She knew that it was not normal to be away from home this late at night and that it was not normal to be sitting in a room with a nurse. She was fidgeting with a lamp cord but eventually glanced up. For an instant her face brightened. I guess I looked like her father.

The children's mother is a blur to me. We were together such a short time and our contact, like that between Mrs. Erickson and me, was limited and strained. Once again I handled the situation poorly. You would think that with repetition I might improve, but I haven't so far. As always, the news weighed heavy on my lips. It lay in my mouth like wet cement. I felt the urge to reach in and manually pry it loose, but somehow it escaped. The words were terse, choppy, and to the point.

Those who think me cold simply don't understand. They haven't had to do it. They haven't had to stare into a family's moist eyes and crush them. They haven't had to crumble a young wife's hopes like desert dirt between their fingers. Each time I do this something inside me dies too. Something warm and caring. Something that simply can take no more savage abuse. Each time is more difficult than the last. This one was especially hard. For as I talked, the young boy continued to sing. He stopped only when he realized his mother was crying.

I would like to say that we were heroic and saved Michael B., but we weren't and we didn't. It would make for a happy ending. But with alcohol such endings are few and far between. With Michael B. there was nothing left to save.

Michael had wandered down a busy road in search of help for his stalled car. The street was dark and he was very drunk. Slowly the stumbling man angled closer to the pavement. Then he turned toward a loud noise. It was a horn. Michael B. was hit by a semi-truck.

I lifted a thin white sheet and pronounced him dead. The man's head had been completely turned around, like the girl in *The Exorcist*. One lung, wrenched from his chest, lay on his shirt. The force of impact had been that great. He was found one hundred feet from the accident site.

After signing the necessary papers, I suggested that his wife not see the body. I had her placed in a quiet room, the one in which we spoke and her young son sang. She never knew exactly how her husband died, about the head and lung and his flying thirty yards. Sometimes the final chapter of alcohol is simply too difficult to reveal. At least it was then. But now, after some time has elapsed, I can tell it. Not directly to the woman, but to you. That is the way alcohol ends. That is why I hate it.

13.

I had time only to hastily scrawl a death note on Michael's chart. I marked the time of passing as 5:30 A.M.

It was getting near the end of my shift; there would be just a few more patients to see. However, as is invariably the case in that gray transition zone between Saturday night and Sunday morning, the time which for revelers is "late Saturday night" but for the religious is "early Sunday morning," in that Star Trek-like time warp that links an old and new week, I see a collection of the city's most pathetic persons. It is as if these fringe humans cannot be outside during any other time of day or any other part of the week. Like Dracula, they must rise from their homes at this specific hour and walk the streets.

During this time I expect the bizarre and am rarely disappointed.

An ambulance crew ambled by with the first of these persons, the arrival of whom had been announced by the distinctive squeak that only an ambulance gurney makes. The driver and attendant were walking slowly, paying no attention to the person they were transporting. And she was paying no attention to them. The patient was an elderly woman with deep lines and creases in her face, the kind that only advanced age can create, like the rock formations in a river valley. Her tangled mane looked like a crowd trying to escape an explosion. A homemade bandage had been wrapped around her left hand.

And the woman was singing. Singing in a high, reedy, inebriated voice while directing a silent accompaniment with her other, unbandaged, hand. This frail, bony appendage made trembling arcs through the air somewhat in cadence with her vocal inflections. Every so often she would entreat the ambulance people to join in. "Sing with me, boys," she said. Then they were lost behind a curtain.

For a moment the air was quiet. The woman was having her temperature taken. With this finished, the music resumed. Two nurses dressed the lady in a hospital gown and laid her threadbare clothing beneath the cart. They took her vital signs—blood pressure, respiratory rate, and pulse—recorded them, and left. Each checked the bedrails before departing.

Since there were no other patients in the E.R., the front curtain was left open. This allowed her warbling voice to carry through the entire department. It wasn't loud but just strong enough to catch your attention, like a dripping faucet. And it had the same disconcerting effect. I moved a bit faster, if for no other reason than to stop the singing. As I entered her cubicle, a somewhat scrambled version of "Stardust" was coming to an end.

"Hello," I said, whirling the curtain closed. "Nice song."

"Thank you," the woman replied, leaning up on her good arm. "I used to be a singer, you know, back in Chicago."

"You didn't have to tell me that," I said, arranging my stethoscope and laying her chart aside, "I could tell."

She smiled as broadly as the rumpled cloth of her ancient face would allow. "You can?" she said brightly. "You know most people think of a sewing machine when I say I was a singer."

"I have a good ear," I said, plugging those good ears with the two plastic prongs of my stethoscope. The instrument, like a long slender insect, put its probes into my head and its head upon her chest.

As I listened, I moved the chilly metal disc around her corrugated rib cage and then, after sitting her up, pressed it at various spots on her back. I was not searching for anything in particular. It was obvious that her problem was localized to her hand. I always begin this way because my stethoscope is the Great Identifier, the doctor's symbol. I am a doctor because I carry one. The cold circle and my warm hands establish an immediate rapport. It breaks the ice. After that things generally proceed well. In this particular case it was difficult to hear anything of medical value anyway. I did, however, catch a throaty chorus of Hoagy Carmichael.

The woman continued to sing while I gently palpated her neck. When I looked into her throat the song changed in timbre, more like gargling, but didn't stop.

Finally I unwrapped the gauze that surrounded her damaged arm. I was expecting another surprise, like the boy with the knife in his hand, and I got it.

The lady's forearm looked like that of a department store mannequin's, the kind that screws on at the elbow. From just below the bend, her entire lower arm was stiff and hard. It reflected the dull ceiling lights. Her fingers were fanned slightly but immobile. It was as if this portion of her body had turned to stone. I touched the dead appendage but got no response. I pinched a piece of flesh and, with a jerk, took the entire chuck with me. Underneath was more of the same. The lady did not notice the missing piece of skin. She didn't flinch. There was no bleeding. She went on singing and directing the string section with her less stiff arm.

I laid her stoney forearm down and recovered it. Despite my best efforts she would not tell me what had happened. She told me about Chicago and her husband the drummer and how he died, but said nothing about her arm. When I mentioned that surgery was in order, she said "fine" and went back to singing.

She smiled as I left but did not break song. Her dusty voice walked me up the hall and was extinguished only after I closed the nursing station door.

The two-man ambulance crew were sitting on a formica counter, chatting with the nurse. One man stood up when I came in.

"Did she tell you what happened?" the man asked.

"No," I replied, sitting on a stool, "all she did was sing. What's the story with her arm?"

The two drivers shared a glance with the nurse. The man who was seated spoke up and rehearsed the details of their visit to the songbird's house.

"We got this call to some sort of rest home, see," he began, "you know the kind of place where the residents all have their own separate apartments? Anyway, we rush over, and the police are already there pushing in her door. The manager had opened the lock but the door wouldn't budge; there was something blocking the way. These two officers are shoving, you know like in the movies," he continued, standing for a better demonstration, "really moving their shoulders into the door, but that thing won't move."

"And all the while," the second attendant broke in, "the old lady inside is singing away. I mean just crooning her tunes like none of this was happening at all. It was her singing that got the manager's attention in the first place. The manager, an old lady herself, says this tenant is all the time waking everybody up with her singing. Only this time when the manager comes to shut her up, the door won't open."

"Finally," the original teller began again, "the cops give a run at the door and bash into the big piece of wood. It moves a bit but then the old lady lets out this Godawful holler." Both ambulance men chuckled. "They had smacked the old bird right in the butt," the teller said, still laughing. "She was part of what was blocking the door."

"But she couldn't weigh more than eighty pounds," I said, remembering the barely existent frame that kept the woman together. I couldn't believe that she was capable of blocking anything.

"Oh she wasn't the only thing on the floor," the first attendant went on, "there's more." Now he sat and finished the story. "Eventually, with all of us helping, the obstruction was slowly moved aside. One by one we slid sideways through the opening. Once inside, we looked around and found everything crammed behind the door, the old lady, the can of soup, and the oven."

"The oven?" I asked.

76

"Yeah, the oven. The woman was on the floor with a big old wall oven right on top of her. ..."

"Don't tell me, her hand was in the ... ?"

"Yes! Yes! That's it!" the driver said, now laughing openly. "This old dingbat had her arm stuck all the way up inside the oven."

"And the oven was on?" I asked, afraid that I already knew the answer. The ambulance pair and the listening nurse all nodded in unison.

"The best we could figure," the original fellow continued, "was that the old lady got tanked. ..."

"There were beer cans all over the apartment," the second attendant interrupted. "I mean it was like she was collecting the things for a contest or something. What a mess."

The first man waited for his friend to finish, then went on as if there had been no break.

"... and after drinking for a while she decided to have a little soup. Anyway, she opens a can of Campbell's, pours it into a pan, and puts the pan right inside the oven, not on the range but in the oven," he emphasized, "so when the soup is done cooking she reaches in to get it but forgets to use a hot pad. ..."

"Ouch."

"I know," the attendant agreed flicking his fingers in the air as if they were burned themselves, "I know."

The second man spoke up again.

"I talked to a neighbor who came out to check on all the ruckus and she said that his lady cooked soup like that all the time. She said everyone, the manager included, had tried to explain about putting the pan onto a burner but nothing got through. The old lady just kept sticking her soup in the oven."

"So," the first man said, crossing his legs and stretching, "she reaches in and gets her hand burnt on this red hot pot. ..."

"And I know the pot was hot," the second man said, butting in again, "because I had to pry it loose from her grasp and it was warm even then."

"I guess," the first man said, losing some of his comic narrative tone, "she must have jumped away and somehow pulled the oven right out of the wall. It was a wall oven, you see," the man said in clarification, "you know, the kind that sits above the range?"

I assured him that I knew what kind of oven he meant.

"The oven and the lady both fall to the floor," he went on, now quite serious, "only her arm is still inside the contraption, glued to this red hot pot, and the oven is on top of her. She is too weak to move the thing and, from the way it is sitting, she can't reach the controls with her free hand either. So there they sit. On the floor. Baking her arm.

I curled my lip and looked at the nurse. She held her stomach and bulged her cheeks like someone who is about to vomit.

"She must have lain there for quite a while" the ambulance medic concluded, "because by the time we arrived she had stopped calling for help and had begun singing. I suppose she finally reached a point where pain wasn't felt anymore. We pried open the oven door and removed her arm. It was well done, I mean cooked perfectly, golden brown."

"What did the room smell like?" the nurse asked, but only because I had been afraid to.

"Just like a dang barbecue," the teller replied, having regained some of his original jocular tone. "It smelled just like a barbecue, like some Western cookout. It was very weird," the man said finally. I had to agree.

This type of thing simply does not happen on Monday afternoon or Thursday night. It can occur only during that Saturday night–Sunday morning lull. During the Kings-X from reality when all rules of sanity are temporarily suspended.

The old woman did not seem to mind that her arm had to come off at the elbow. "Do whatever you want," she said during a break in "September Song." That was the last time she spoke to me. She would answer no more questions. She just kept singing. I was amazed at the number of tunes she knew. She never stopped singing and never repeated a song. One right after the other, she warbled out old melodies, none written within the past twenty years. She went off to surgery amid a rousing chorus of "Hold That Tiger."

Then I called upstairs and caught the second surgeon just as he was leaving. I explained to him about the oven and the singing lady. He concurred that it was a "different" story and graciously consented to stay and take care of the problem. He suggested that we send the lady right up. He also mentioned that the boy who held up the hospital pharmacy had survived his operation.

When we heard the good news, a wave of surreal elation flowed over the entire staff, like warm saffron honey. It lit a common spark of hope and faith. A burst of honest satisfaction painted everyone's face. Even I had to smile. I promised myself that I would shake the miracle surgeon's hand. The man who had operated with no blood. That was like driving with no gas. But then, luckily, some rides prove to be all downhill.

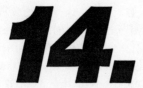
14.

I had time for one more patient and, as if on command, that patient arrived. To no one's surprise, the man had consumed a bit of alcohol, and, as a result, became involved in an auto accident. He had banged his head and sustained a large cut on his right forearm. A thorough inspection showed that to be the extent of this lucky fellow's injuries.

The policemen who arrived with him said that the man had driven his car into a pole, demolishing both. Had he not been drunk, and thus very loose, his problems could have been much worse.

The fellow was sent to X-ray for films of his head, neck, arm, and pelvis; all, fortunately, proved negative. That meant he had no broken bones. He asked if the pictures had shown a concussion. I said no.

It is interesting how pervasive some medical misconceptions can be; a few have become almost universal. One of these is the mistaken notion of a concussion. Most people are surprised to learn that a concussion, like almost anything else but a fracture, does not show up on X-ray. (A fracture, incidentally, is the same thing as a break. Many persons think these are two separate entities. They say, "Thank God it's only fractured; I thought it was broken." They are two words for the same thing. A concussion is a symptom diagnosis. It is any neurological complaint following a blow to the skull. For instance, a person, like this man, is struck on the head. Perhaps he is knocked unconscious, perhaps not, but afterwards he does not remember what happened, or he has a headache, or he cannot move an arm, or whatever. This is a concussion. Some are more severe than others. This gentleman had a mild one.

During my examination, while he was in X-ray, and all the way back, the injured man kept asking the same three questions, over and over: "Where am I?" "How is my wife?" and "Do I need stitches?" After one round would finish, another would start. This reaction is called "perseveration." A brain acts like any other injured tissue. It swells. This swelling can cause a series of cerebral short circuits, one of which is recent memory loss. Thus, despite being answered each time, the same questions were being asked.

I reread the fellow's stack of X-ray films and was again relieved to find no bone breaks or evidence of other pathology. Satisfied with my diagnosis, I requested the nurse to set up a suture set, a tray upon which are sterile instruments used to repair cuts. As she was doing this, the questions continued; "Where am I?" "How is my wife?" and "Do I need stitches?" As before they were answered, "You are in the hospital," "You need stitches," and "Your wife is fine," which she was. Although involved in the same accident, she had miraculously escaped unharmed. I brought her to the bedside in hopes that seeing his wife might jog the man's memory. It didn't. With the lady sitting almost beside him, he asked, "Where am I?" "How is my wife?" and "Do I need stitches?" I sat down to repair his arm.

Local anesthetic was drawn up and injected around the cut. The supine man jerked slightly at the initial pain but quickly forgot his discomfort and repeated the trio of questions. I answered without stopping my hands. A package of suture material was opened—these days it is made out of plastic, the subject of another common question—and grasped the needle with my sewing instrument. As I began to sew, the sensation in the patient's arm must have rewired another circuit. He added a fourth question to his repertoire. Staring down at his arm, he asked, "Am I getting stitches?" "Yes," I replied, holding the dangling thread directly before his eyes, "you are getting stitches." He looked around the room, "Where am I?" he said again, followed by "How is my wife?" "Do I need stitches?" was dropped. I answered this new set of inquiries for ten minutes. By then his wife, having sat dutifully and silently all the while had had enough. She rose from her seat and stormed to the man's side. The frustrated woman brushed a clump of hair from her forehead and shouted, "I'm fine, Goddamn it, I'm fine. I-am-fine."

She patted herself on both arms and then down her sides in an attempt to indicate somatic integrity, then she grabbed her husband's face and aimed it at her own. "See," she said in triumph, "I'm okay."

With a startled look the man said, "That's good, that's good."

I touched the wife's arm and she let go of her spouse's head. She apologized and returned to her seat. The patient turned back to me. "Where am I?" he asked, as if nothing had happened.

"You're in the hospital."

"Am I getting stitches?"

"Yes."

"How's my wife?"

I looked at his wife and she looked at me. We both burst out laughing. I had to set down my needle holder and stand. She had to leave the room. It was difficult to wipe my face without using my sterile-gloved hands but I did, then sat and finished the repair.

The wife and I enjoyed another laugh back in the hall as I peeled off my gloves and explained to her about head injuries and the need for close observation. We both agreed that a night in the hospital was in order. The arrangements were made and she walked to the admissions office.

It was 6:30 A.M. and nearly time to go home. I sat in the nurses' station and propped my feet on the counter. All of my bones ached, even the small ones that few people know about. I had a constant drone in my head like flies at an August picnic. My mouth was dry, as if someone had lined it with cheap cotton. These were familiar symptoms. I got them every night that I worked. They are all cured by sleep.

I finished my final chart and walked away to change clothes. As I was leaving, the car accident man sat up and asked, "Where am I?" I was in no mood for another round of three questions and would have ignored him had it not been for a changed quality in his voice. This last question had lost the singsong, broken record lilt that marked all his previous quizzings. This time his words contained a sense of intelligent anxiety. He sounded as if he really wanted to know. I walked back to the bedside and said, "You are in the hospital."

"Oh," he replied, acknowledging for the first time his presence anywhere. "What happened to my wife?" he asked, craning around as if finally comprehending that he had begun the evening driving but now did not appear to be doing so.

"She is fine," I repeated for the umpteenth time, but added hopefully, "You were in an accident and got hit on the head. Your wife wasn't hurt. She is here with you. She stepped out for just a minute but will be right back." I smiled into his frightened face. He seemed relieved. Then he looked at the baseball seam in his right arm.

"Did I get stitches?" he asked in the queer way people do when looking at an old photograph, taken way back when they were thin and had hair.

"Yes, you did," I answered truthfully, "I fixed a cut on your arm."

"I see," the man replied, rotating his appendage as if it were not his, admiring the plastic railroad track. "I'm sure glad I wasn't here for that," he said with genuine relief, "I hate stitches."

I couldn't strifle a laugh. The man smiled, not entirely certain what he had said was so funny. I chuckled all the way down the hall and into my office.

There I removed my blood-spattered shirt and pants, the green ill-fitting scrub suit that keeps other people's fluids off my body. I put on my regular clothes.

With a few minutes to spare, I lay down. We keep a small bed in the office for such occasions. I imagined that I would only close my eyes for a few seconds, just until my relief man came. Then I was hot and sweating and the pillow had been knocked to the floor. It was 7:30. The new doctor had laid his things in the corner and left me alone. He said I looked as though I could use an hour's sleep.

It took a few seconds to reorient myself. The walls seemed unfamiliar and the sun was shining at an odd angle. I ran an open hand through my hair and across dry lips. I pressed three fingers into the bony bridge of my nose and exhaled. I had been dreaming about the boy in surgery with no blood. I dreamed that he had died. White and screaming. It took some thinking to realize that he had actually survived. Then I remembered the pharmacist. Perhaps he had been the one in my dream? But hadn't I chosen him to live? Hadn't he survived his operation also? With a twitch in my stomach wall, I realized that I had no idea what had become of my friend. I had been so relieved that the one picked to die had lived that I just assumed the one picked to live had not died. I resolved to call surgery immediately.

Checking my wallet and keys, I walked out of the room. There was a new flurry of activity at the end of the hall. Nurses were walking briskly into the code room. I saw the tail end of a paramedic. He was bent over and pumping. Without thinking, as if in response to some animal survival instinct, I whirled away and went out the back door. I could tolerate no more. I would call the hospital and ask about the pharmacist when I got home.

There are no windows in the Emergency Department. The reason for this, however, has never been clear to me. As it is, the E.R. is like a Las Vegas casino. In it you lose all sense of time and day. The hours pass, marked not by any shift in shadows or change of temperature, but by the imperceptible creep of two pointed clock hands. Without rest or fail those two spears circle their numbered dial, around and around, like a stone grinding wheat, pulverizing day after day and life after life, turning both into an unrecognizable mixture of bland, tasteless powder.

I don't know if this forced timelessness is by chance or design. I suspect a bit of both. No one wants outsiders peering in, but a bit of fresh air and a slant of sunshine would be nice on occasion, especially when daybreak has touched rose to the Eastern horizon. For some reason just a glimpse of this quiets an inner turmoil, like an atmospheric tranquilizer, and allows me to face another day.

With a few quick steps I was out the rear door. The morning desert air hit my face with a bracing primordial rush. The air knew nothing of pharmacists and robbers or of blood and no blood. It remained cool and complacent, tingling the world with gossamer stillness. I swam through this exhilarating brilliance until I found my car. It was covered with a thin layer of dust. A windstorm had blown through during the night. When one emerges from a place without windows, the outside weather becomes a regular surprise. I brushed the flecks away and opened the door. With a turn of the key, the engine sputtered to life.

Soon I was moving with the radio on. I rolled down my window, putting my face into an artificial breeze. It felt good to be away from the hospital. But most of all it felt good to be alone and not to have to make any decisions for a while.

15.

There are drawbacks to Emergency Room work that affect not only working hours but nearly every other one as well. The schedule is odd as people get sick at unusual times. Meals are missed because it is hard to break for lunch with your hands inside a child's chest or when converting a lethal heart rhythm. And your sleeping suffers. In short, any biological clock is checked at the department door.

I find myself awake during "Farmers' Report" and asleep while others watch the national news, or vice versa. Many nights, after my family has gone to sleep, I will wander the house, sensing creaks and analyzing dull shafts of street light, synchronizing my heartbeat with the kitchen clock. I listen intently to the silence, hoping to fuse with its mortal sameness, wishing that some deep night rhythm or distant celestial pattern will carry me away. But then my mind intervenes and stops the meandering. It intervenes with questions about my patients, things I should have done but didn't or things I did but shouldn't have. It pricks me with yesterday and reminds me of tomorrow. It knows that soon I will be back. Back in the windowless cavern where sick people come. It knows and my body suffers.

My stomach is chronically confused. Often I will find that it is 7:00 A.M. and realize that I have forgotten to eat for the past day. A string of nights will pass during which I won't eat at all. Five or ten pounds will be shed from my waist, but in a week it is all back. My belt is in perpetual motion, defying some scientific law.

Add to this a carved-up social calendar and the jumble is complete, the confusion total. Yet, in some larger scheme, these are but minor psychological aberrations, more in the realm of irritating distractions, annoyances, gnats on my mental elephant. They are not nearly, I have come to appreciate, as important as the fears.

The Emergency Room has generated in me a vast array of real and imagined fears, a pharmacopoeia of diverse and interesting misgivings. The problems with meals and sleep are erased by time, but the fears stay. They have become a bridge between days and a tie around weeks, like an unwanted emotional epoxy. They have, in a bizarre twist, become one of the few things upon which I can depend.

They began as twinges, small embryonic feelings of compassionate apprehension. "I'm glad that didn't happen to me," is what I said in the beginning. I had not as yet made the transition to "That might happen to me." But then the incidents seemed to grow larger, more mentally demanding. The self-questions became keener and the self-answers less acceptable. Until there were no answers left. Then they were fears.

As a result of my job I have come to view the world as an inherently dangerous place, an environment in which, if I am not ever vigilant, some manner of harm waits continuously to befall me. Even the mundane has become spiteful. I have developed a disquieting general dread that makes nights darker and shadows longer. I have bred an envious resentment for abandon.

These fears come from my patients, my Emergency clientele, and their things. People and their machines. Or more correctly, the people and what their machines have done to them.

I have been forced to accept the fact that man and machine don't mix. At least not when the people are drunk and their machines wheeled. Or when men are tired and their machines sharp. Like oil with water, hands don't mix with saw blades. Or eyes with welding arcs. Or wrists with roller skates. Or thumbs with broken glass. The list is long and continues to grow, as people invent new machines or discover novel ways to harm themselves with the old.

I have become intimidated by commonplace objects because I have seen, in abundant supply, the distinctly uncommon things they can do. Everyone has read at one time or another about a man mowing his lawn who dies when spinning blades hurl a stone through his heart. Or you hear on the news about a baby that choked to death on a pop-top ring. Someone is always falling down stairs, or off the roof, or drowning in the bathtub. Every year a number of persons get shocked while adjusting Christmas tree lights. Butane cigarette lighters explode. So do cars. For me these experiences are multiplied manyfold. They have grown until they seem like the only experience.

And there always looms, like raindrops over a picnic, the spectre of the largest machine, the mechanical sword of Damocles. The machine that demands the most respect and receives the least. The machine that orders, like an oriental potentate, a homage of human lives. The machine that people think in, love in, drink in, and play in. The metal contrivance that they use and abuse. The machine which, in return for all the disrespect, extracts an enormous payment, a pound of flesh splattered on the road. The machine that kills. Your car.

I have developed, over and above my many small worries, a strong aversion to driving. I have seen so much damage that a deep distrust has developed, like a mother's fear of polio. It is not the goosebump ripple I feel when watching an awkward child whip past on a skateboard or the tongue-clucking expectation while watching a man round his woodwork past a jigsaw blade. These are smaller fears, mere trepidation in contrast. The larger terror is born of severed limbs and missing heads. Of legs ripped from lifeless bodies. It is a mortification born of policemen and their icy humor. And of undertakers with a solicitous grin.

One day these fears, the great added to the small, will finally become too much; they will pass a point of critical mass. One day they will at last become too strong and, like a crippling spinal disease, they will paralyze me. In the end, the image of a mangled child or brains in a bucket seat will become so vivid and the fright so real that it will bolt my front door and seal the windows. It will weight my bed blankets with rusty iron anchors, while underneath I will lie still and quiet, trapped in a bell jar of my own design. Trapped but safe. Safe in knowing that I will see these things no more.

Martin L., on the advice of his agent, took out additional life insurance. Although healthy, and despite what most would have considered adequate coverage, he listened to the man's pitch and dutifully signed. Martin L. was a family man. And as the salesman said, "You just never know." Obliging as always, Martin L. fulfilled the peddler's promise.

The actual policy, an impressively lettered paper with monogrammed leather case, was placed in the family safety deposit box. Six months later the document was removed.

Martin L. proved a liability on the company books. They received but forty dollars in premium payment yet paid $30,000 in claim.

While driving home from a small mountain town where his wife and children were spending the summer, Martin became drowsy. He pulled off the road at a rest stop. After an hour's nap he felt somewhat refreshed. He took a sip of water and used the restroom. Checking his watch, he started the car engine. He did not, however, flip on the headlights. Martin had spent all afternoon in a direct sun, driving the family water ski boat. He had taken two turns in the water himself. His legs ached. He had a sunburned back that tingled each time he moved in his seat or shifted gears. So the omission of front lights was understandable.

The returning father had gotten a late start home. Not having seen his family all week, he had stayed an extra hour. This set back his arrival to well past midnight. He had been up early that morning, too.

Without lights, Martin's car slipped unnoticed onto the freeway and he began a run down the outside lane. Had there been a policeman or another motorist nearby, perhaps Martin's lack of illumination would have been noticed and the situation corrected. But there was no one in sight. Except the truck.

The semi driver also did not know Martin's lights were out. He didn't know Martin was there at all. Until it was too late. Until he felt a bump and saw the small car flip. Until he saw the tiny auto roll four times and burst into flame. The stunned trucker jumped out of his rig and ran as near to the orange lapping wreckage as heat would allow. Then he could only stand and stare.

The conflagration soon attracted a passing patrolman. And then another. They consoled the grieved truck driver and, when the twisted metal mess was finally cool, arranged for it to be removed. What was left of Martin they placed in a plastic bag.

With their city home empty, it took the better part of a day to locate the dead man's family. By chance a neighbor noticed the lawmen on the lawn and told them about the summer cabin.

Although uncertain of an exact address, the authorities managed to sort through faraway vacation homes and eventually found Martin's. When she was told of the accident, Martin's wife burst into tears. What I experienced to a lesser degree, Martin's wife then suffered acutely. From that day on she never drove again. Or, for that matter, rarely even left home. A friend took her to the funeral. She was white knuckled and trembling all the way. Her anxiety and grief became focused on cars. If she avoided the large machines, maybe things would be better, and the hurt less intense.

Martin's eldest son was seventeen. He, along with his mother and sister, shared equally in the windfall insurance money. Money from the "just in case" policy. Money for which each person made plans. Martin's wife became even more depressed when her son revealed his. He was going to buy a car.

The night I spoke to Martin's wife I said that I understood, although in retrospect there is no possible way that I could have. As I talked, her face went flat and firm. Dead. Like her son. I'm still not certain if she heard my voice. She made no reply and her eyes never blinked. They remained cold and steady like lamps that had long been switched off.

Martin's daughter had a different reaction. She wanted to talk. So I listened. She was the one who told me about her father and the car fire and the summer home and the police coming to the door. She spoke freely about the accidents and the insurance money. She said that her father's funeral had been closed casket as, she assumed, would be her brother's.

But her face belied its true emotion. The girl had sunk, understandably, into an abysmal state of denial. She told me that she was a cheerleader at school and that she didn't think she would mind being an only child.

The son's accident was a near Xerox copy of his father's. He also met a truck on the freeway. His car flipped but didn't burn. It landed upside down. A group of bystanders were recruited to right the belly-up auto. Then the firemen went to work. With large shears they cut through the door and extricated the nearly dead boy. Two men became ill. They bent by the roadside. Other cars slowed but were motioned on by a flare-waving policeman.

Most people don't appreciate the size of eyes. With lids covering the upper and lower portions they appear to be small and almond shaped. You forget that they are actually round, like golf balls.

When I saw the son's eyes they were round. They were round because he had lost the lids. The insurance money car had been a convertible and on its first roll-over the boy's head had been scraped along the pavement, removing scalp and forehead. The young man's body arrived at the Emergency Room. The missing skin was left at the scene.

Despite the loss of face and hair, the boy's heart was still beating. But soon, mercifully, it ceased. Since that night I have discussed this particular anatomical problem with a number of plastic surgeons. None could come up with a good answer. Had the teenager lived, they said, reconstruction would have been enormously difficult. But he didn't live.

Unlike his father, the son had not been tired. He had been drinking. The smell of partially combusted alcohol permeated the death room for almost an hour after he was removed.

I have no way of knowing what occurred inside the mother's mind following her second loss, but it must have been dreadful. Some final plug was pulled, a Rubicon crossed. She still had a daughter but that was not enough. I saw this woman,

Martin's wife, the dead boy's mother, one other time. Then she too was staring up at me from a hospital cart.

Four empty pill bottles were found by the mother's bedside. There were different dates and different doctor's names on each container. The pills had been laid in a long row and swallowed; she started at one end and worked her way to the other. There were three pills left when she collapsed and was discovered on the carpet by her daughter. A garbled note was left on the nightstand.

The nearly comatose woman had her stomach pumped. Blobs of decomposing pills were removed. They proved, however, to be no match for the larger, more potent blobs that sailed through her bloodstream and lodged in her brain. I put the lady on a ventilator and watched her wheeled upstairs. Later that night I watched her wheeled back downstairs in a green zippered bag.

I should have spoken to the daughter then but I didn't. I simply could not bring myself to do it. In my confused state of mind I believed that had I talked to her again about cars and death, she too would have died. An invisible chain needed breaking and I was desperate for a way to do it. I purposely stayed at a far end of the building until she was gone, led out by a nurse, picked up on the ramp by an aunt. Then I crawled back.

For me, episodes like this can easily distort reality a good long time afterward. Events, as they did then, can become too complex and confused. Usually this happens when I treat people who have mixed with machines. It all makes me wonder who is in control. And how to stop it.

Perhaps shunning them, not talking or even thinking about them will make the killing cease. If I refuse to recognize their existence will I see no more teenage boys without eyelids? Will it stop daughters from watching their families fall like metal ducks at a carnival stand? Or by not looking, by not carefully analyzing, am I missing some subtle link? Some hidden clue? Some association or rule by which this craziness can all be understood? I don't know. I don't think I will ever know. Now when I get into my car and begin driving, I look in the mirror and see myself with no eyelids and with a ventilator to take my breaths. I see my wife fingering a cache of Seconal bottles. I see my daughter twisting a braid of hair and humming to drown out the nurse's voice that is saying everything will be all right and that her aunt will be there soon to pick her up.

I slow down. I brake. I watch for cars up every side street. Then a car full of teenagers speeds by. Or a man without headlights. Or a girl drinking. They all seem oblivious. They are talking and laughing. Not watching. Don't they know there are trucks on the road?

Suddenly I am screaming. Hurling my voice at the darkened headlights or the tipped can of beer. But no one can hear me. I keep the windows rolled tight. There are so many accidents and so many daughters that I have learned to keep my windows shut.

Even if I could grab those drivers and push my warning into their faces—Please Slow Down! Be Alert! Don't Drink—even if I could shake them, I know they wouldn't listen. They would, despite my best efforts, still maintain that eyes are oval and covered with lids.

part two

SUNDAY

1.

I spent most of the day sleeping, waking sometime in midafternoon to the distant sound of televised basketball.

It was an NBA playoff game I had planned to watch. The room was hot and stuffy. A thin layer of sweat had accumulated on my skin. It made my body briny and damp. The bedsheets smelled of this same coming summer heat.

I walked out on the patio and waded into the swimming pool. Warm, sun-heated water rose slowly from my knees to my chest, dissolving that coating of night-worry and humid day-sleep. It seemed as though I had woken once that day already, and I had; this made it difficult to guess what day it was. A newspaper was folded by the side of a lounge chair. It had been left there by my wife Sandy. I pushed up out of the water and padded over. Just below the headlines was the day. It was still Sunday.

For a while I forgot about work. I let the sun dry my skin and blank my mind. Heat sunk deep into tired muscles and weary bones. When beads of sweat appeared on my face, I toweled off and wandered out to the garden. There, amid my carefully nurtured vegetables, I picked an occasional intruding weed and generally took inventory of the sprouting plants. Despite its being just early spring, the desert growing season was approaching its middle. All my produce had to be in by the first of July. After that, the backyard would become a blast furnace, shriveling everything alive. I had just that morning read an article about snow in the Rocky Mountains and a freeze in Kansas. Our temperature was 93 degrees.

Then I wandered back to the pool and added chlorine tablets, poured in a steamy cup of acid, and scraped drowned bugs from the surface.

My family had been to church that morning. I could

tell because everyone was still dressed in their best. Shannan, my eleven-year-old daughter, had on a skirt, which in itself should have tipped me about something being unusual. I know they had asked me to accompany them to the service, and I know I said no thanks, that I was too tired. I don't actually remember any of this but my wife tells me it happens that way every time I work the Saturday night shift. That I could not remember the church invitation did not bother me nearly as much as not remembering the drive home or going to bed.

My wife and I talked while we read the paper. I lay on the couch gazing at the ceiling. The sun had passed its zenith and was casting longer and longer shadows. Food smells were wafting from the kitchen. Then I jerked up. The shadows were gone and dinner was on the table. I had been napping. I swore then and there to quit the Emergency Room. I do this three or four times a week, if for no other reason than wanting to wake up only once a day like everybody else. It seemed like three separate days already and it was only Sunday afternoon.

As dinner progressed I began to grow edgy. My motions became quick and rapid, like a movie running fast. I looked out the window a lot. Perhaps I am being dramatic, but this must be, I have concluded, the sensation an athlete gets before a big game. The closer it got to 6:30, game time, time to return to the hospital, the more tense I got. Soon I couldn't sit still. The meal was a disaster, as it always is when I am in this state. Food went down grudgingly and left a veneer of nausea in its wake. I could not tolerate casual conversation. Social Studies homework or problems with the pool man just didn't seem important. I snapped at Sandy and glared at the children, unfairly of course, but I couldn't seem to help it. My family suffers right along with me, perhaps even more so.

Finally I had to leave the table. I tried reading a page from an Isaac Singer book, something that generally calms me, but could finish just a few lines, and even those didn't register. When I had read the same sentence five times, I set the book down. I played a phonograph record but that only made matters worse. The sound seemed loud and out of synch. I shut it off.

98

Finally it was time to leave. I kissed everyone goodbye and promised to call. More often than not I don't, but I want my family to know that I am thinking about them. I have told my wife that soon I will cut down my hours. For her that can't be soon enough. She has started making this point in passive ways. When I came home late one night last week she threw up her arms and said, "Take my jewelry but don't harm the children." Even the dog barked at me.

Clouds had gathered during the afternoon, bringing a cool tint to the air, something very noticeable in the kiln-baked Southwest. A taste of moisture tinged my lips.

The sky was now dark and foreboding. A black hat of clouds had lowered over the city, leaving just a band of silver around the edges. Soon even that was gone, and with a report of thunder, the drops began to fall.

Rain in the desert is like rain no place else. Each individual particle seems larger and appears to fall faster than you have ever remembered. It must be because downpours are so infrequent that they seem so intense. And so much water accumulates on the ground. Soil here is more like cement than dirt. It doesn't soak up a cloudburst, it repels and then propels it. I sailed as much as I drove to work.

At last, lunging through one final sidewalk-straddling lagoon, I splattered two fans of rooster tail spray into the hospital parking lot. Picking what appeared to be the shallowest puddle in which to park, I stopped the engine and turned off the radio.

For the next half-minute I simply sat and listened. Only with a concerted effort did I shake myself from this rudimentary meditation. It was seven o'clock. I ran across the parking lot and stepped onto the electric mat; the Emergency Room doors slid open.

"Back again?" the receptionist asked, grinning at me from across her desk.

"I just can't get enough of a good thing, Vi," I said,

pushing open the inner swinging doors.

"You can't fool me," the woman replied, turning back to her typewriter. "You're just a glutton for punishment."

I left the waiting room and Vi's clattering typewriter and was once again inside the Emergency Department. The difference was like night and day. It was sudden, sobering, and instant. Outside had been active but reserved. People were seated in tiny cliques, all rehashing details of the misfortunes that brought them there. Parents were standing behind children in wheelchairs. Each youngster had a baggie full of ice plopped on an injured appendage. There were people in bathing trunks and others in three-piece suits. A solitary man peered over the top of his magazine at a pretty woman across the room. A child stretched for an out-of-reach button on the candy machine. The waiting room could have been any place, a bus station, a party, halftime at the football game; people were people, and things were calm. Inside the swinging doors it was different.

2.

The first thing I noticed was a change in smell. Nearing bed one, I caught a familiar odor. It permeated only the immediate area but was unmistakable. It clung to the air like dog hair on wool. An acrid tang stuck in my nostrils for many minutes after. It was the stench of bloody vomit.

At the bedside our day doctor and a crop of nurses were attending a pale patient, the source of this nasal insult. Initially I only saw the sick man's shoes. His feet dangled at imprecise angles, like two strangers waiting for a bus. Then I caught a glimpse of his face. It was sallow and moonlike. A large-bore tube, the size of a small garden hose, had been passed through his nose and into his stomach. This internal pipe was evacuating a steady stream of reddish brown muck. The patient's gown and the nurse's hands were covered with the same gritty sludge.

One staff woman was flushing iced salt water down the nasal tube. This was supposed to freeze the man's stomach and cause his leaking vessels to contract. She alternately filled a huge syringe with freezing water from a metal pan, pushed this frigid mixture down the tube, waited for it to settle, then sucked everything back out again. A second nurse was busy with two intravenous lines. The only free person was flitting about filling the air with propellant aerosol droplets, which abruptly changed the omnipresent smell to scented pine.

I stopped in the station to see if they needed any help. A clerk said no but thanked me for asking. I went back to the doctor's office and put on my scrub suit.

With a change of clothes the transition was complete. As I walked from the tiny office I felt as though I had never left. It could have been that morning again when I had first awakened. The same wave of apprehension and surge of insecurity immediately returned. It was as if these feelings had been hidden in my pastel hospital shirt, just waiting for me to put it back on.

My beginning routine was the same. Just as on the previous night, the departing doctor gave me a rundown of current patients and mentioned a few interesting things that had occurred during my absence. I noticed that his shirt was splashed with hemorrhagic effluence but, like the air, it too had been plastered with freshener. The man was a mess but smelled like a forest. Not unexpectedly, my associate was again anxious to leave. Tonight his closing dissertation was short. He had no smile or parting comment. He walked away quickly, shedding his damp shirt while still in the hallway.

I leaned over the counter and checked the bleeding man through a window. He was our most ill patient and had been placed in the bed with the best view. His feet were still askew and his face ashen, but the tube seemed to be clearing. At least now there was more water than blood being pulled back. Still the nurse kept plunging and removing. She would do this until the ruby fluid became totally clear. Which it finally did. Slowly the red turned to brown, then pink, then streaked, then nothing. At last there was just water, down and up. The bleeding had stopped and his stomach was empty.

There was replacement blood being processed in the lab which he would receive in the ICU. We would transfuse him, then wait. Wait for him to bleed again.

With the stomach bleeder gone, there were now five people for me to see, three patients left from the afternoon shift and two new ones whose fresh charts a nurse was depositing in the rack. I rubbed both palms together in a silent movie representation of "going to work." My mind eased into gear as I walked to the chart holder.

Perusing the lot, I chose the simplest first. I needed to get off to an easy start. From a wheelchair parked in the hall, I delicately manipulated the misshapen wrist of a forty-year-old man. He seemed as embarrassed as hurt. At first he said he had fallen off a ladder. But during my exam a red-haired boy stuck his head in the door and asked if this meant that the skateboard would have to go. The father said no, that accidents just happen. Then I asked him again what had happened. He told me about watching his young son easily mount a wheeled board and glide across the driveway cement. He told me about forgetting how difficult it really was and about how fast those new plastic wheels went and how much farther he had grown from the ground. I assured the fellow that this sort of thing was very common.

The fallen skater went to X-ray with a cold pack on his wrist. The bone was later set and cast. He left with a white arm hung in a sling. The eleven-year-old asked if he could be the first to sign the cast. The father raised his plaster hand as if to clunk the boy's head, then hugged him close and laughed. The man's wife took his good hand and they all left.

Another of the remaining day patients was a woman with vaginal bleeding. The departing doctor had seen her only briefly, deferring the pelvic exam to me. After I saw her, I swore an oath to repay him for this favor. Because he hadn't mentioned anything special about her other than that she was a little overweight, I put off seeing the woman for a while. I would wait until I had cleared up some other problems. I wished later that I had not done this.

The final "leftover" was a young man who had been injured in a motorcycle accident. A large gash ran the length of his forehead, the edges of which formed ragged flaps like pennants in the breeze. There were a number of small rocks embedded inside, pieces of stone wrenched from the pavement. I knew there was no skull fracture underneath because I could see the bone directly. This main laceration was surrounded by an audience of smaller ones.

His chest and back were glistening red, like fine USDA steak. Both areas had once been upholstered with skin but were no more. He looked like a tree with the bark ripped off. This condition is known as "road rash." Only it's not a rash. The red, the part that looks like a rash, is really what is under skin. Road rash comes from falling off a motorcycle and skidding down the street, leaving your skin behind. Although very tender, the denuded regions must be thoroughly cleansed. This process is painful. Despite large doses of narcotic medication and tightly bound hands and feet, these patients always put up a God-awful fuss. They scream and thrash while a nurse scrubs their body with a wire brush.

This man's feet and hands had been badly scraped also. I counted his fingers and got ten, toes nine. He had not been wearing shoes. One leg was strapped in a metal splint. The calf and knee were fine but the thigh was shaped like an "L", as if someone had added another joint. I pressed on the fellow's abdomen and listened around his chest. His insides seemed to be all right. There was a trace of blood in his urine, not at all uncommon after such a tumble, but I could find no major source of life-threatening trauma. I did see a helmet under the table. It too was gouged and scraped. Had he not been wearing that head protector he would have been dead.

The man had been drinking. This combined with our painful steel-bristle-cleansing, made him very combative. Even in the firmest leather restraints, he thrashed about wildly, cursing in a loud and forceful voice, displaying a prodigious physical strength and an imaginative vocabulary. Between cursing spells he bit at anything that moved. Finally a bedsheet was tied around his head. The biting stopped but the swearing continued. "Maybe we should have tied the sheet around his mouth," I said.

As the body stripping progressed, like scouring paint from an old house, we were all privy to an entirely new realm of language.

By motorcycle standards his were only moderate injuries. I see less extensive ones but rarely more severe. The bad ones, of which there are many, either go directly to an operating room or down to the morgue, mostly the latter. A good many people have bikers to thank for their organ donations. Dead cyclists, especially those who ride without helmets, provide an invaluable supply of hearts, kidneys, and other organs. Around the hospital these vehicles are known as "murdercycles."

I made certain that proper orthopedic and plastic arrangements had been made, then closed the curtain to the skinned man's cubicle. This only slightly muffled the young man's vulgar tirade. His abusive language was an insult to me, the staff, and anyone present, but at least he was coming clean.

With the motorcycle man as background noise, I shifted to the new patients. I picked up a chart and read the name, then looked at the age. I had seen a young girl in bed four on my way down to the motorcycle man and this was her.

When I pulled the curtain open, she didn't seem to notice. Lying in bed, indeed taking up so little of the bed that it almost looked undisturbed, was a very pretty young lady. Her hair was blond and short, well combed, with a red barrette clipping one side away from her ear. Makeup had been expertly applied to the youngster's face, giving an impression of one somewhat beyond her stated years. Below the bed was carefully folded clothing, a pair of faded blue jeans, a red sequined top, wooden heeled shoes. I took an opportunity to scrutinize her before she saw me. And I didn't like what I saw.

There is an art to medicine that cannot be taught. Certain feelings come only with intuition and experience. One is the ability to recognize, any other evidence to the contrary, a seriously ill individual. It is imperative that a physician know, or at least suspect, when a well-appearing person is sick, just as it is important to recognize when a theatrical person is only acting. I decided from just a look, from an unlearned gut reaction, that no matter what this girl's lab work disclosed nor what I found on physical exam, this was a very sick person. It was something in her eyes.

The young woman was lying sideways in bed, both hands beneath the sheet and pressed to her belly. Her knees were curled up, a position not unlike that of poor Mr. Erickson. But Mr. Erickson had come in with his wife; this girl was alone. There was no one in the bedside chair. No one to hold her trembling hand. No one to say that things would be okay. And no one to wipe perspiration from her streaming brow.

The chart said that she was sixteen, although I suspected less. I asked when she was born and she said "1966" but quickly sputtered, "I mean 1964, sorry."

Either way I had a problem, a constant dilemma facing Emergency Department physicians: what to do with minor children. They are old enough to get themselves grievously injured or become seriously ill but not old enough to sign for their own medical treatment. On these unaccompanied teenagers we always try to get parental consent. Unfortunately, this can sometimes lead to delays in treatment or unnecessary suffering on the child's part.

We have standard consent forms that parents can sign and deposit at the hospital. Once completed, these sheets allow us to treat the children when their parents are away. But most people neglect to return the forms. Once a child is well it is difficult to imagine him sick again.

Yet, despite legal statutes and parental consent, if children need quick treatment, they get it. Unfortunately, that was to be the case with this girl. She was young, very sick, and had come in alone.

"How are you?" I asked while lowering the head of her cantilevered bed. This sinking motion elicited a moan. The question elicited nothing. "What seems to be bothering you?" I continued.

The child opened her dry lips and muttered a reply. It was inaudible and had to be repeated. "I've got an awful stomach ache," the girl said a second time, then clutched tighter at her abdomen. Even the effort of talking hurt.

"I see," I said, and proceeded to run through a stock series of questions aimed at locating the exact site and nature of her problem. She said that she had vomited twice in the past hour, but had not had diarrhea. She said she felt feverish. I glanced at the temperature our nurse had taken. It was 102 degrees. She said that her pain had begun the night before and was slowly getting worse. Now it was constant.

Next I asked her a more general variety of questions; included was a query about her menstrual history. With this, the young lady's responses suddenly became very short and abrupt.

She would not say when her last period had occurred nor when the next was due or if they were regular. Forgetting her pain for the moment, she actually sat up. "That sort of thing is not important!" she volunteered, her face flushed with fever and anger, "the problem is my stomach." My exam indicated otherwise.

I apologized for upsetting her and she settled back down, once again lying sideways facing me. I lifted away a covering sheet and pressed slightly on the child's legs. They straightened some but not as much as I would have liked. To palpate her abdomen I had to walk around the bed and reach across her pretzeled torso. I began at the outer edge of her solar plexus and worked circumferentially inward. It did not take long to localize the source of pain. It was in her pelvis. And not just the right side, as one would expect with an appendicitis, but the entire area. Each time her lower region was touched, the youngster winced and tugged at my wrists. She tried to conceal her distress but could not. I moved my hands away and pressed below her rib cage. I pushed the skin down, then let it suddenly fly back up. She let out a yelp. This is called "rebound tenderness." It meant that the membrane lining of her abdominal cavity was inflamed. It meant surgery. And I suspected what kind.

I replaced the top sheet. Although it wrenched at deep visceral instincts and firm promises to emotionally separate myself from my patients, I felt as though I were tucking in my eleven-year-old daughter. The girl was curled as my daughter does, only not for sleep but from pain. I touched her shoulder and said that things would be fine. I said that the lab would be in to draw some blood and that an X-ray was in order. Then I asked about her parents. I knew this was the kicker, the 64,000 dollar question.

The child immediately forgot our brief bond of intimacy. "My parents aren't here," she said with a jerk. Her face swung around and her body straightened. Then she cringed and stammered, "Look Doc, this is nothing serious. I just have a stomach ache. Once you give me a shot I'll be fine. Besides," she said, forcing a grin, "my folks are out of town ... they're on vacation and I don't know where to find them . . . they're in California or Oregon somewhere. . . ." Her final words shot out, as if fired from a gun. She had become extremely agitated. This only confirmed my supposition about the cause of her problem.

"If not your parents," I asked before departing, "a boyfriend maybe? Did anyone come with you?" A blaze of fury filled her eyes. Both hands grabbed fistfuls of sheet. Tendons stood out on bony forearms. Her lips quivered. "No," she shouted with mounting anger, "I told you I came in alone. . . . Do you know what that means? It means no one is with me. No parents! No boyfriend! Nobody . . . I came in alone. . . ." Her last sentence was softened somewhat when she had to double over and brace her stomach to keep it from exploding. Two pearly tears the size of schoolyard marbles welled in the outer corner of each eye.

"Don't worry," I said, reaching out and holding her hand, "we will take care of you and make things better. And we won't call your parents." This wasn't true, of course, but it was what she wanted to hear. She managed to say "Thank you."

The child needed surgery; her mother and father would have to be notified. I had lied, but for a reason. Right now I required this girl's trust and complete confidence. I needed time to complete her lab work and to find a surgeon.

Occasionally a certain amount of truth-stretching must take place. I understand this grates against many persons' sensibilities, especially those who write articles for national magazines about honesty between doctor and patient. But so be it. Sometimes this type of prevarication is necessary, and not only with children. Besides, lying had gone on by both sides. If that girl was sixteen I was General Grant.

Back in the central station I looked at her chart again. My next concern was about her name. I doubted that she had given the right one. "Susan Smith" just did not ring true. I was facing a very complex problem.

"Linda," I said corraling the youngest nurse I could find, "I need your help." I thought the sick girl might relate better to someone closer to her own age. The lady I chose was a new nurse just out of training. She was twenty.

"What can I do for you, Dr. Seager?" she smiled.

"Do you see the patient in bed three?" I asked, tipping my head in that direction. From our angular vantage we had a view of the girl's body but only part of her face. We could both see that she had balled up again. We could also see her partially obstructed face held over a plastic bucket. She was vomiting again too.

"Yes, I see," the new nurse replied, "she looks ill. What can I do to help?"

"I need you to go in and speak with her. I think the child has had a butchered abortion and is afraid to tell anyone. Her uterus is exquisitely tender and I noticed a spot of blood on her gown. When I questioned her about her parents, her menstrual periods, or asked about a boyfriend, she came unglued. I thought she was going to hit me." The nurse moaned in genuine disgust and pity, a pervasive combination of emotions that infects the Emergency Room. "Why do people do these things?" it says. The feeling becomes stronger when patients are young and their predicaments precarious.

"She won't divulge a thing to me," I continued. "Says that her name is 'Susan Smith' and that she is sixteen years old. I'll bet," I said, looking directly at the new nurse, "that if you approached the subject and showed her some affection (something that I suspected had been in short supply recently) she might let out with the truth. It's extremely important, Linda, that I get an accurate history. Any assistance you can give me would be greatly appreciated."

"I'll try," the nurse said, somewhat frightened by the task but grateful for the trust, and then she walked out to see Susan Smith.

My intercessor was gone but a few minutes when a frightening problem reared its head. From small footprint flattened drips of water in the hallway I knew that the outside storm was continuing. I also knew because the lights weakened. For just an instant everything was brown, then gray, then black. It was like going blind in slow motion. With a deep basement grunt, motors whirred again and the color change reversed. Finally the lights again beamed brightly. Electrical wiring, I am told, is like a fighter: it can take only so many punches before going down.

3.

If alcohol is King Annoyance in my Emergency Room life, then drugs are Crown Prince. The E.R. is one of few places where narcotic medication is kept and dispensed, and like a house fire or an auto wreck, this attracts certain people—those persons whose physical well-being depends upon that medication.

Addicts come in every shape and size, need-gratification being no respecter of class, age or profession. And all have a story aimed at getting their drugs. Most are simple. A few could open on Broadway. I spend a good deal of valuable time listening to the anguished tales of mid-twenties males who cannot bear the agony of their turned ankles. I grudgingly face elderly women's apologetic requests for a Percodan prescription refill because their "doctor is out of town." I am asked to give nervous housewives Valium. I fend off the terrified blunt appeal of thin young women staring down the barrel of opiate withdrawal.

As do most physicians, I have a federal drug number and thus am legally licensed to write pain pill orders. Hence I have become a focal point in the battle between substance, addict, and law enforcement. For the habitué who must scavenge in the street, I am the legitimate connection, a port in his strung-out storm, the candy man in coat and tie. I can write a legal fix.

In our Emergency Room there are two boxes full of 3 by 5 cards, each with a name and short blurb printed on it. The original box, a recipe-sized metal container with hinged chrome top, was filled long ago, and we are well on our way to filling the other. A third will be needed soon. These boxes contain the alphabetized names and aliases of persons who repeatedly come requesting drugs. As we change doctors frequently, and work irregular shifts, it is unlikely that any one physician will recall any specific patient. But with a cumulative file, any doctor can check a suspicious story.

Reading through the file is entertainment enough for an entire evening. Randomly selecting a card will invariably produce an interesting story. One gentleman signs in with severe flank pain. He brings with him an irregularly shaped stone, obtained from God knows where, and says that he has just passed this object in his urine. Anyone who has had or knows about kidney stones realizes that the pain is almost unbearable and that narcotic medication is definitely in order. Addicts know about kidney stones. They know, in addition, that there is a special X-ray study which will document the presence or absence of a renal rock. It is called an intravenous pyelogram or IVP. Basically, a radiopaque (impenetrable by X-ray) liquid, Renografin, is injected into an arm vein, it circulates freely, finally accumulating in the kidneys, causing them to "light up" on X-ray film and outlining small obstructions, like stones. Doctors order this test on persons they suspect of having ureteral calculi. Most addicts know about IVP's too. At least this man does. He claims to be allergic to the dye.

I must admit, one of the better-thought-out stories.

I actually saw this fellow once and immediately recognized the trap. I had read and commented upon his card many times. I felt that I knew him. As I went to do my exam, I was actually nervous. It was like meeting a movie star. Or some remote relative whom you had heard about all your life.

I parted his curtain with unfettered anticipation. We exchanged hellos and he was "on." I leaned back and listened. It was like hearing a favorite bedtime story. "Uh-huh," I said, as he described the burning rip in his side. I touched the area in reverent silence. "I see," I went on as he told about giving birth to this hard, round object. "Allergic to IVP dye? What a shame!" I said in reaction to the punch line. Then asked if I might take a look at the stone. He presented his hand and opened it slowly, as if transferring a very valuable gift. He rolled the object into my palm with flair and finesse. It was his crown jewel.

I held the ball up to the light and inspected it closely. Moaning softly, in an imitation of stoicism, the man bent slightly and clutched his flank. When I pointed out that the stone had little bits of pocket lint stuck to it, the moan changed to a gasp. He looked horrified. Now it was my turn to act. I excused myself to answer a not ringing telephone. Before leaving, I set the stone back on the bed. The fellow looked like the cat caught with a mouthful of parakeet feathers. When I returned he was gone. And so was the stone.

Addicts know a good deal about other laboratory tests too. They know that blood in the urine is also a tip to kidney trouble. Just a drop of hemoglobin in a large container of urine will turn this key test positive. When this was pointed out to me, I began kneading the fingers of all suspicious persons when they turned in their specimen. More than once a positive lab result has coincided with a drop of blood from a punctured thumb.

Back pain is another favorite. And it is a good one too. Not as clever as the kidney stone scam but very popular nonetheless, especially among the over-thirty crowd. There is no reliable way for me to dispute this story nor any readily available test to disprove it either. When someone says his back hurts, I am obliged to believe him. There is, however, one drawback to this seemingly infallible approach. Back pain is not worth the heavy duty drugs, the industrial strength pain relievers. Ten Tylenol with codeine and a muscle relaxer is the most anyone can expect. It takes a good many E.R. visits to live on that. Still I am certain that I have aided many an addict over a temporary dry spell by treating their "back hurt while lifting."

These are but two highlights in an almost endless list of patient complaints. There are numerous others: migraine headache, regular headache, an almost migraine headache, an almost regular headache, an old industrial injury, an old war injury, a new industrial injury, a new war injury, a low tolerance to pain, no tolerance to pain, an allergy to pain, a religious belief against pain, and the same tag line comes with every story, like a caboose on every train—a death-like reaction to every known drug except Demerol.

Fighting the drug battle wearies me. It also spends a good deal of insurance company money (read: "your money").

But these are not its worst effects. Because of my continual sparring with the chemical cravers I have come to suspect everyone with pain, real or not. I find myself questioning the legitimate stories and lowering my sights as a reliever of genuine misery. Some people really do hurt their backs or have actual kidney stones. The patient has become an adversary, a hostile witness whom I must trip in his story. I have switched from doctor to prosecuting attorney. Which story is real? Who is faking? How did this injury really happen? Tell me more! Where is the pain exactly? Be more specific! Had I wanted to be a lawyer I would have gone to law school.

As I do with so many other upsetting emotions brought on by the Emergency Room, I fight this accusatory posture and try to be sympathetic. But it is difficult—especially when the man with the terribly painful ankle grabs his prescription and runs for the pharmacy. I hate feeling that I have been had.

And I hate frustration. The kidney stones, ankles, and backs are distasteful but not gut wrenching, not like the lives that drugs waste.

Before I could see the next scheduled patient, I was hustled off to bed two. Lying there was a vomit-spattered seventeen-year-old girl. Her head was turned to the side and her mouth was open, the way people's mouths hang open when they are asleep. She was dribbling yellow partially digested food onto the sheet like a broken rain gutter. Her clothing was stained with the same mustard-like liquid. Friends had brought her in and literally dumped her at the waiting room desk, their car running all the while. Then the friends left. Two security guards and one technician rescued the slumping girl. One stood under each shoulder while the third pushed from behind. The lady's feet dragged the whole way. There were scuff marks leading from the hall to the bed.

The receptionist handed a paper bag to the nurse. She said that the people who brought the girl left it up front. It was full of pills and pill bottles.

Our first order of business was to stabilize the patient. A nurse cleaned out her mouth with a plastic suction hose. Now the yellow vomitus filled a wall bottle instead of leaking into lungs. Another nurse started an intravenous line and hung a bottle of salt water. This not only would give us access to her circulation but would also afford me the opportunity to force fluids through her kidneys. More urine would be produced and more drug cleared. At least theoretically.

I reached for the intubation tray, a flat metal stand containing instruments for putting tubes into bronchial pipes. I selected a hose about eight inches long and as big around as my ring finger. With the flip of a metal blade the girl's open mouth was invaded and her tongue lifted out of the way. A small bulb shone down her throat. There were blobs of food and pill obstructing my view, I called for more suction. A vacuum stick was inserted in the now crowded mouth and the organic litter removed. Then I could see her windpipe.

The breathing pipe was greased for easy passage and aimed at the twin target vocal cords. I pushed it down but quickly removed it. "Suction!" I shouted as the child's mouth again foamed with vomit repulsed from an irritated, raw stomach. Just a touch to the back of her throat had been enough to set off the reflex. Amber sludge once again slid down her cheeks and onto the bed. A large hose quickly scrounged the gastric juices, making a sound like the last bit of water going down a bathtub drain.

Then I tried again. This time the insertion was swift and deep. The tube entered the trachea, sliding up to the hub. I inflated a small-tip balloon—this kept the tub in place—then stood back as another bolus of vomit blew out of the girl's mouth. With her airway occluded I was no longer worried that the oxidizing eruptus would find its way into her lungs. This final blast was cleansed while artificial breathing began. The girl had not flinched during all our intraoral manipulation. She was sinking into deep coma. She did not blink when I grazed her bare eyeball with a cotton swab.

Next came the large stomach tube. A thick hollow snake, its hind end stuck into a huge, water-filled beaker, was stuffed in the child's nose, pushed down the esophagus, and passed into her stomach. Immediately a gallon of clear water was run in and let right back out. This was essentially the same thing that had been done for the bleeding stomach earlier but this water was not iced nor was it allowed to linger internally.

The returning fluid was dusky brown and spotted with multicolored pills, the same colors that, in intact form, now sat on the station counter in a paper sack. It took six flushes of water before I was content that no more drug fragments were forthcoming. I ordered one more batch of liquid sent down the tube. It was to contain a large amount of charcoal. This ground-up briquet dust would adsorb any bits of chemical left in recesses of the teenager's gastrointestinal tract. Hopefully any hideouts would be collared by the soot and carried away, rather than absorbed and transported to the brain.

With this done, I ordered lab work and I.V. medication. I gave Narcan and glucose, my standard comatose fare. The sugar did nothing, but the Narcan helped. Some. The child made a few feeble respirations and wiggled a foot. I was facing a dreadful therapeutic challenge. There were not only narcotic drugs on board, which I could antidote with Narcan, but other more insidious substances as well, most likely barbiturates, tricyclic antidepressants, hallucinogens, and God knew what else. For these I had no antidote. I told the nurse to give regular Narcan injections and sat down to decipher what pills the girl had taken.

There is a book, the PDR or *Physicians' Desk Reference,* which lists all the drugs made by American pharmaceutical firms. It contains information about proper dosage, common side effects, and the symptoms of overdosage. It also has color pictures of the pills—I turned to this graphic section and began to match the glossy ones in the book with the solid ones in the bag. As near as I could tell, the girl had taken Percodan, a narcotic pain reliever; Valium, a muscle relaxer and mild tranquilizer; Triavil, a drug given for depression but one that can be extremely lethal when taken to excess—it makes the heart beat funny, then stop; phenobarbital, a drug used for seizures but

116

from the same family as Seconal, a potent sleeping medication; and finally the ever-present Quaalude, another sleeping pill. But not just any sleeping pill. This was Quaalude the media star, number one on the drug top forty, the hip head buzz word, the name that commands immediate attention and knowing smiles. Quaalude is a brand name for the chemical methaqualone.

It is not that Quaaludes are more dangerous or more potent than most of the commonly misused drugs, or that they produce any better "high." They have just received better publicity. Television networks do hour shows on Quaaludes. They are always making the papers too. "Underground Laboratory Discovered," "Plane Load Intercepted," "Street Value of Six Million." They are the talk of the high school and college campus, where they are affectionately known as "ludes" for short.

Perhaps it is the name that has brought about the mystique. Maybe something in the sounds of "Kwaaaluuudde" calms an inner beast or is in synchronism with an untapped biorhythm. Or maybe, like Jello-O or Levi's, the name just caught on.

"Ludes" are interesting to talk about but not so to take. Especially in any quantity and with other drugs, which this girl had done. For her, the interest was staying alive. She was facing death—the ultimate high.

I administered another medication to combat a rapid heart rate, which I assumed was precipitated by the Triavil, in strong doses a cardiac irritant. Her pulse slowed somewhat after the shot and her general condition improved.

I was attacking the pills and their problems one at a time, treating them in the order in which they were arranged on the desk. I had done what I could with the Percodan and the Triavil. I passed over the phenobarbital; there was nothing to do for them right now, except wait and pray the girl didn't die. The Valium did not warrant specific treatment. I suspected that alcohol was on board as well and was proved correct when a high blood level was found. It was in the intoxicated range. I only hoped that PCP was not involved. This drug is a nightmare. It is known as "angel dust" or a dozen other street names. Originally developed as an animal tranquilizer, it is a drug that makes people do very strange things. Like pull their eyes out. Or jump in front of trains.

We had done all we could for the moment. I walked to the central station and made phone connection with our internist then called for a respirator. I was glad to see the somnolent girl head upstairs. I don't like watching young people die. They are too near my own age. The fact that someday I will also die, suddenly becomes very real.

The internist phoned me later and said that he had examined the girl and was making plans to dialize, a word that means hooking someone up to an artificial kidney and leeching poisons from their bloodstream. He called again an hour later and said that the dialysis had been cancelled. He said they would have called a code but all the necessary people were there anyway. He said that the child's heart had stopped beating after her circulation collapsed. The doctor stopped by on his way out and thanked me for all I had done. He gathered what information we had about the girl; her name, the fact that she was a high school junior, her insurance number, and the fact that she had taken the pills on a dare. Information obtained by looking through the dead girl's purse and from a comment made by one of her "friends." Then the internist left for home and the young girl went down to the morgue.

It is easy to pontificate about kids and drugs, especially after a head-kicking incident like this one, but we see just as many adults who are near dead from alcohol or who have OD'ed on their own brand of medication. And it is not limited to the public. The hospital staff is vulnerable to the allure of pills and booze also. They too understand the comfort of a needle.

When I was an intern and rotating on the oncology floor, I began to notice that pain shots for a good number of our terminal patients did not seem to be working. These shots were for persons whose bodies were riddled with huge sheets of malignant cancer cells and whose pain was caused by snapping bones and crushed organs. After deciding that all the medication could not be ineffective and upon hearing similar stories from the other physicans, I launched an investigation. It was soon discovered that some of the night staff had been injecting themselves the potent narcotics and shooting the patients with water. While the help were in a stuporous haze, the dying faced their pain alone.

It makes you wonder. What have we done to ourselves that would allow people to do these things? To even think them? When dealing with drugs and their human toll, I recall a definition of the E.R. given to me when I was in medical school. Someone said that the Emergency Room is like that little mesh grid that sits at the bottom of a sink. It is the lowest place in the area and traps all the junk before it falls down the drain.

After treating that pill-ravaged child I was in no mood for the next patient. And his complaint was one that set off my fireworks display of drug emotion. His chart said simply, "ear ache," but I recognized his name. He wasn't in our Betty Crocker recipe file, but in my personal file. A private customer, if you will. I had seen him before at another hospital a few years back. I knew that I could dispose of him quickly.

The first time I saw this gentleman, he had also complained of ear pain. I remembered his ear, red and raw; and I remembered his name, John Jones. I remembered, at the time, speaking with other doctors who had also seen him, and deciding upon how he got his ear to look so bad. We concluded that the man unwound a coat hanger and poked the sharp end in his ear, then scratched and scraped until the canal was hamburger. We surmised that he was very careful and got lots of practice because his drum was never touched.

The first time I saw him I ordered only eardrops and explained that there was local anesthetic in them. He refused the prescription and demanded Demerol. I said no. He left in a huff. That had been three years ago; now he was back again.

Fortunately our second encounter was brief. Had he pressed me and asked for Demerol as he did before, I was prepared to eject the creep bodily. But it never came to that. Perhaps he saw the fire in my eyes, or maybe he really did remember. Because when I entered the room and said, "Remember me?" he looked at my face, glanced down at the floor, and said, "Yes I do." Then he got up and walked out. I threw his chart all the way across the nursing station. It rained paper and carbons up and over the desk. I apologized to the ward clerk, who picked it up. She said that she understood.

No sooner had I collected my thoughts and most of the strewn paper when my young nurse appeared. She had spent the intervening time talking with "Susan Smith." "You're right," was all she said in passing, then she took a seat at the far end of the room, facing the window, legs squeezed tightly and hands folded. Finally she broke. With her face buried in her hands and her neck bent, she wept. I left her alone. I would speak to her later, when she was more composed, after I had seen the final-day leftover, the woman with the vaginal bleeding. And I nearly got to see her too. I got as far as the cubicle curtain when a nurse took my arm and led me out to the ambulance ramp. Once there I assisted an extremely ill man from a rescue vehicle. That man was Walter T.

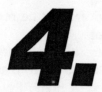

4.

Walter T. had served during World War II and, like other young men far from home, he found love. At war's end, along with a shattered leg, he brought home an Oriental bride. I met both Walter and his bride the night Walter took ill and came to our Emergency Room. I met them the night I was best man at their wedding.

Walter T. sailed from San Francisco early in 1943. He had enlisted immediately following the shock of Pearl Harbor and was sent to Fort Leonard Wood, Missouri, for basic training. There, despite his expressed desire to fight, he stayed an entire year. There had been some confusion with his paperwork, they said later.

With files at last in order, a call to the front came. And out Walter went. He landed on one of those South Pacific atolls that, until the war with Japan, neither he nor anyone else even knew existed. For the next eighteen months Walter and his unit hopped from obscure island to obscure island, slowly creeping toward Japan. Those islands had funny names; but after half of his friends were dead, suddenly the names didn't seem so funny.

On one of these palm-dotted stops, the kind that Ezio Pinza would later sing about, Walter stepped on a land mine, a calling card left by the retreating Nippon Army. It was a reminder that war is not nearly as romantic as some writers can make it seem. And a reminder that legs are not really very well attached.

Walter was separated from the lower part of his right leg but luckily held onto his life. The man standing to his direct right was never seen again. Walter was evacuated back to a humid, open-air hospital where a long and painful convalescence began. However, it was not as painful as it might have been, nor as long, because of the tender nursing care that he received in that thatched frond hospital. From Sumi.

Walter married his nurse. They shared a unique bond that only wartime settings can afford. He was far from home and sick. She had no home and was scared. A bomb from one of the planes had seen to that. Sumi cared for Walter and kept him from dying, both from his injuries and from loneliness. He quickly fell in love—or what he thought was love. It was really, another woman would later explain, just simple gratitude. This second woman explained that to Walter just before he abandoned Sumi and married her.

It seems that Walter had not anticipated the problems of an Asian wife. I suppose one does not think about language and customs when he finds love far from home. Away from any prior reference. In a place where rifles are being shot at you and where young men lay dying at your feet.

After ten years, forgetting love, rifles, and dead young men, Walter divorced his transplanted bride and married the woman who had explained the difference between love and gratitude. I never met the second wife, the explainer. She wasn't at the wedding. In fact, she didn't come at all during the night. The night I kept Walter alive.

Walter T. finished the job the Japanese had started. He drank himself to death. After his leg was injured, he had turned to alcohol. Despite the attentive care of his native nurse, there were still many long, uncomfortable hours to fill. Alcohol kept him company and killed the pain. During the time they were together, however, Sumi managed to keep the problem in reasonable control. But once she was gone, he took to heavy drinking. Very heavy drinking. His second wife, the one who knew so much about love, also knew about alcohol. She was an alcoholic too.

The last months of Walter's life had been spent in and out of hospitals. He contracted cirrhosis, a hardening of the liver, brought on by his alcohol abuse. It made him very sick. It made him turn yellow. Blood pigments, no longer broken down by his diseased liver, were deposited in his skin. He took on the permanent shade of a ripe lemon.

Then his muscles wasted. His abdomen began to swell. He became mentally confused. Poisons jacketed his brain.

Once Walter became ill and turned yellow and began to shrink away, his second wife left. This time she did not explain about love and gratitude. Had he felt better, perhaps Walter could have reminded her. But he never felt better.

It was during his first bout with severe hepatic failure that Walter learned the real definition of love, gratitude notwithstanding. Having heard of his troubles, Sumi came back. Walter's doctor told me that she took her ex-husband home and nursed him. Again.

With the aid of a friend, Walter divorced his second wife. As a result she received most of what Walter had left, what he hadn't drank away. But he still had insurance from a policy he had purchased before joining the service, and he wanted those benefits to go to his real wife. Plans were made to remarry Sumi.

That was when I met Walter, the night before the second wedding. The night that his heart failed and nearly stopped beating. The night his lungs filled with fluid. The night through which he had to live: he was getting married in the morning.

Walter was pulled from the back of an ambulance. He was breathing rapidly and perspiring profusely. His face was swollen and yellow. We put him on a gurney and wheeled him into bed two, next to the girl with the hacked abortion. He required immediate treatment. I would worry about his chart and paperwork when they got there later.

The ambulance driver said they had been called to a home by an Oriental woman. She told them that Walter had done this sort of thing before, having just been discharged from the hospital last week for the same problem. They said the woman was on her way and they gave me the name of Walter's doctor.

Walter could not speak; it was all he could do to breathe. Toxins in his blood were strangling his brain. He could form no conscious thought. I lifted his eyelids. Both eyes were blue and yellow. Like two flags. There were no white parts left.

Veins bulged in his neck like fat, well-fed worms. They vibrated with each heart contraction as shock waves rippled through stagnant blood. Blood was backed all the way to his feet.

I propped the man and listened at his chest. His lungs were full of gurgles and sloshes, like water in a half-filled bucket. They were dripping wet.

Walter's heart, like failing hearts in general, made a galloping sound instead of the more familiar "lub-dub." His chest sounded like the Kentucky Derby. His stomach was too bloated to examine. Ankles, although skinny, were also bogged with water. The man's body was full and tense like a child's balloon. Walter was drowing in his own internal river. No place was left unfilled. Even his eyelids were puffy.

A nurse started an intravenous line. This was easily done. All the man's veins protruded like huge subcuticular ropes. I ordered medication to be given. A heavy dose of diuretic, medicine to make one lose water, had a transitory effect. For a few minutes Walter's respirations softened and he sweated less. But he soon lapsed back. A nurse informed me that his blood pressure was beginning to waver and take episodic dips. I doubled the water-extracting preparation and administered the larger amount. Nothing. It was apparent that medication alone would not be enough. In an effort to pool part of this ubiquitous fluid in the large fleshy extremities, to keep it from the lungs, I had rubber tourniquets placed at the top of Walter's arms and legs. Gravity would pull water down, away from the chest. Intravenous morphine was given and large amounts of oxygen administered. Finally Walter began to hold his own. We had temporarily stopped his death slide.

I took a break and went to phone the icteric man's doctor. I was certain that Walter's dreadful condition would prove to be no great surprise, and it wasn't. During our conversation, the other physician retold Walter's rocky medical course. He told me about his patient's losing fight with the bottle and about his second wife, whom, he added, had not seen Walter since the day he took ill. I explained to him what we had done and he concurred. For the moment it was agreed to leave things as they were. Then he told me about Sumi and the wedding. I promised him I would do my best to keep the man alive for his ceremony. The doctor said he would check back later. I agreed to make arrangements for Walter's hospitalization and to call immediately if anything changed, which I strongly suspected would happen. We exchanged good-byes and hung up.

From the window, poor alcohol-soaked Walter looked like Humpty Dumpty. He teetered in bed like a huge painted egg; round, yellow, and unaware, a human ship afloat in his own ocean. I knew that, like the fabled egg, Walter was going to take a great fall. Then Sumi arrived.

The woman was tiny even by Oriental standards. I spoke to her sitting down. She said she knew how ill Walter was and thanked us for what we were doing. I told her that I knew about the wedding and said that we would do everything possible to get her husband-to-be out of danger. It did not seem proper to offer congratulations. We shook hands and smiled, then she made her way to the admissions office. I wrote some instructions to the nurses regarding Walter's care and handed them to the ward clerk, who tubed them upstairs.

For the moment I forgot about fluid, weddings and the lady with the vaginal bleed and looked for my distressed young nurse. I found her back in the lounge. She had stopped crying, and with the exception of two faint black streaks of runny mascara, her face was clear. She had a half-filled cup of coffee and a smoldering untouched cigarette.

"Well?" I said, sitting beside her.

"You were right," the nurse repeated, only this time in a voice not nearly so charged with emotion. "The girl is fourteen and her boyfriend, a worldly man of sixteen, got her pregnant. She told her prince the good news and the next day he disappeared. No one has seen him since. She called the boy's house and his mother said that he had gone to visit an aunt in

Texas." With that the white-capped woman took a long, powerful drag on her ash-laden cigarette, then crushed it out in a paper cup. It hissed in a drop of water. "I thought," she said twirling the sizzling butt between two red enameled fingernails, "that the girl was supposed to go visit an aunt?" Then she gave me a sarcastic smile. Even this early in her career, the disease of E.R. cynicism was taking root and beginning to flower.

"Times have changed," I answered, knowing full well the burden of anger this young nurse was being called upon to bear. "Please go on."

"Anyway," the woman continued, her voice now totally devoid of any feeling, "she didn't tell her parents, but she did tell an older girlfriend ..."

"And this 'older girlfriend' just happened to know a place. ..." I answered, riddled myself with the same street-wise sarcasm, the kind of give-a-shit toughness that slum kids learn early but that comes to E.R. personnel late.

"Exactly! Some clinic downtown that she can't remember the name of did the job for her yesterday. She said she didn't feel very well afterwards but thought that some pain was probably normal. But the burning never got better, only worse. Now she's scared," the rapidly maturing nurse added, taking a sip from her lukewarm coffee. "She knows that something has gone wrong."

"Did she or her friend call this place and ask for help?" I asked while running through my mind all the abortion clinics that I knew were operating in town.

"They both called and got a recorded message. It said the office would be closed until Monday and would they like to leave a message."

"There wasn't anybody on call?"

"Nope."

"No one to answer the phone even?"

"Nope."

"You mean this clinic just abandons their patients over the weekend?"

"Apparently so," the nurse answered, equally as disgusted as myself. "I guess they figure anyone smart enough to realize they are sick will be smart enough to go to an E.R." The young woman uttered this final line with almost complete moral insensibility. She was a fast learner. She knew that there was a whole department full of patients and to cry over each one would take the entire shift. So you cry over none.

"I imagine," I added, standing to leave, "that she gave us a wrong name? Somehow 'Susan Smith' just doesn't make it."

"Most likely," the nurse agreed, getting up to follow. "She wouldn't budge on her or her parents name. But I took her purse while she was in X-ray and I will go through her wallet. I'm certain there will be something in there that will give us a name."

"That's good, very good," I said as we both left. I felt like the Artful Dodger commending young Oliver Twist on his stealthy work.

"She made me promise not to tell you any of this," the old-new nurse said as we entered the hall. She bit her first fingernail and walked ahead of me.

Again with an animal-like groan, the lights and electric fans heaved a tired sigh and sputtered. Everyone froze and looked to the ceiling. We were very much relieved when the bulbs glowed and the fans blew again. The only person who seemed not to notice was the young nurse who had betrayed the trust of a fourteen-year-old girl.

5.

I returned to the nursing station and had the ward clerk phone our gynecologist. She spoke to the doctor's answering service. The teenage girl needed surgery, and he would have to perform it. I was grateful to my neophyte nurse for the valuable information she had collected, even if it did mean sanding away a layer of her humanity to do it.

With so much time expended upon Walter and my conversation about the aborted girl, other things had backed up considerably. That blond child with her rotting uterus was stuck in my mind and nothing seemed able to dislodge her.

Again, I tried to see the woman with the vaginal bleed but was stopped before I could get out of the nurse's station.

For the first time that evening the paramedic phone, a short wave field-to-hospital line, beeped. Its irritating shriek demanded and got my complete attention. I sent the nurse down to check the bleeding woman then lifted the receiver and pushed the "talk" button. "This is Dr. Seager, go ahead," I said. From the other end a scratchy voice gave me the rundown on a woman who had been shot. Our connection was very poor; it took three repeats before even rudimentary information was transmitted. The firemen were inside a home with screaming children and a grown man moaning in the background. I was able to piece together only a skeleton history and the patient's initial vital signs. Then the line got clearer—the children must have been moved to another room—and more information was exchanged. Appropriate medical measures had already been taken. I had nothing to add. I said that we would be prepared for their arrival, which they said would be in fifteen minutes.

In that abbreviated and tense interim I checked with my relay nurse who said that the bleeding woman seemed to have stopped bleeding and that she would hold for the moment. We barely had time to ready the code room before the paramedic entourage arrived. With an efficient flurry, the wounded woman was deposited in the code room bed and hooked to our life-support system.

The lady was conscious but only barely. She jumped when stimulated by pain, a firm skin twist over the sternum, and moaned in response to her name. But nothing else. Her blouse was quickly torn away and silver-dollar–sized monitor leads glued to her chest. She was breathing with the aid of a plastic tube already inserted down her throat. When a connected black bag was compressed, her chest rose.

Just below a wingspread of ribs and very near the center of her body was a single bullet hole. It was no larger than a dime. There was a dark ring of powder around the edge. A gun had been fired point blank. I searched but could find no exit hole. The bullet was still inside.

The transfer sheet was signed, not unlike an invoice, and the paramedics thanked us. They were in a hurry, having already been summoned on another call. One fireman mentioned in passing that the woman's wound had been self-inflicted. The result, he said, of a heated argument at the home.

Her legs were encased in inflatable vinyl pants. They had been put on by the medical attendants and filled with air. Like a dam, this pressure helped keep blood away from the less essential legs and near the vital head and heart. Thus blood pressure for these central organs was kept high enough for them to function properly. The "mast suit" would be removed in the operating room.

In prearranged routine, nurses, laboratory technicians, and X-ray people skillfully performed their specific tasks. A catheter was inserted in the woman's bladder, filling a bag with warm, blood-tinged urine. An artery and a vein were punctured and blood removed. X-ray films were shot of the chest and abdomen. In a large central vein I started an additional fluid line by inserting a long needle just below the patient's right clavicle and threading a small tube into the pierced vena cava. I ran the line in, feeding it like rope, until the tip was just above the woman's heart. This would allow me to administer large amounts of fluid or medicine should they be needed. Also, ac-

130

curate venous pressure readings could be taken from this deep visceral location.

When I had finished, her X-ray films were ready and some initial blood work was back. In addition, our on-call surgeon was on the phone. Before I spoke to the other doctor, I held the black plastic X-ray film up to a view box and saw why there had been no exit wound. A bullet was lodged in her spine, directly between the fourth and fifth lumbar vertebrae. The bones themselves looked fine. The missile must have cut only soft, defenseless nervous tissue. I asked if anyone had seen the patient move her legs; everyone said no. When I thought about her eggshell-delicate spinal column being slammed by a steaming bullet, I doubted if she would ever move them again. I gave these details to the calling physician, took operating room orders from him in return, them hung up.

Self-inflicted damage is a difficult problem for me to face. It generates competing emotions and sorting them out isn't easy. When you are trained to value human life, it is hard to deal with those who treat it in a cavalier fashion. And yet a disquieting admiration surfaces also. When I think of death and its sobering reality, it is difficult to imagine anyone choosing it voluntarily. In some bizarre twisted logic, suicide takes a sort of courage, I guess. I still wonder, though, why these people don't just get on a bus for Cleveland, take a new name, and start all over. But, as a friend pointed out, suicidal problems are usually inside and you can't run from those. Those kinds of problems can escape only through bleeding holes or into a deep bottle of pills.

There was a time, during my respecting-their-courage days, when I felt sorry for the victim, and I still do in a way, but not nearly as strongly or exclusively. I have sat alone with a twenty-eight-year-old man, his eyes cloudy and placid, blood clotting on his temple. I have cleaned up after a thirty-year-old woman who had swallowed two hundred No-Doz capsules— and dozed permanently. She vomited so many times that her room had to be scrubbed out twice. And I have attended spent elderly persons who could not face another lonely day, the refuse of modern miracle treatments, a cruel reminder of life prolonged beyond its biological end point.

After all of these I still harbored a sympathy for the deceased. I empathized with their problems and tried to understand what drove them to such drastic action. But that view proved to be shortsighted. Soon another side was presented. The other side arrived with a sixteen-year-old boy. Now every time I deal with suicide or an attempt, I view things differently.

A nurse said that the bleeding woman and her husband had been arguing. (The nurse had quickly cornered a family member in the lobby while we were initiating therapy. She then filled me in.) The patient had accused her husband of having an extramarital affair, something, the relative said, that occurred with some regularity, but this time the man vociferously denied it. The wife did not believe him. She ran across the room and pulled a revolver from the nightstand. Before anyone could move or speak, she had driven a bullet into her own gut. Why she did not point it at her head was puzzling. Perhaps she just wanted to scare her mate and did not realize what awful damage a missile to the abdomen could wreak. The couple's two small children had been standing in the doorway while all this happened.

Although maudlin, it is nevertheless true that no person is an island. A suicide victim, by his capricious act, always hurts those who love him. For instance, what effect will their mother's insane play have upon those two children? Will they imagine, as children frequently do, that they are to blame? Will the husband ever forgive himself for driving his wife to such destructive action? Will the crippled woman, should she survive, exercise a guilt-fueled dominance over those who were in the room that night? Will she spin about the house in a motorized wheelchair, a living symbol of her family's shortcomings? Will the others be able to go on if she doesn't survive? Was this hideous stunt just a way to get even? To get attention? To gain control?

I never asked these questions or any like them until I saw that sixteen-year-old. He changed everything. He gave me the needed insight.

A teenage boy took a liking to a pretty and popular girl in his high school class. After months of hesitation and self-castigation he finally screwed up the courage to ask her out for a date. And to his amazement she accepted. She was a cheer-leader and he was a nobody. They went out one time, maybe two. She found him unusual and interesting, but too intense. He always wanted to talk about God or the planets or Sylvia Plath. She wanted to talk about the homecoming game. Unschooled in emotional etiquette, the boy brashly pressed for more serious involvement. Repeatedly the girl refused and summarily dismissed him one evening over the phone. His appeals quickly became bellicose and bizarre. He phoned continually. "Marry me or I will kill myself!" he stated finally. "I never want to see you again!" the girl retorted with equal sincerity.

She had other, more normal suitors, who made less strenuous demands, she said. Totally demoralized, the young man made one last sobbing plea. He was turned down flat. Perhaps it was then that something burst. Maybe it had happened a long time before. No one ever knew.

Thirty minutes after their last phone conversation, the girl's doorbell rang. She answered. It was the boy. He was dressed in a blue three-piece suit. She had never seen him in anything other than jeans. He had meticulously combed his hair. He looked like someone going to a wedding or a funeral, which, in a way, he was. The young lady was startled but invited her friend in. She could not imagine what he was going to say or how she would respond. She never got the chance to discover either. Instead of entering, the boy produced a shotgun from beneath his coat. Both barrels had been sawed off and fit underneath a suit jacket. He raised the gun to his head and blew the entire right side of his face away.

Paramedics drove the boy to our E.R. with a towel stuffed in his head. He still had a faint heartbeat but that quickly slowed and died. That was the first time I felt rage over suicide. It was also the first time that I really understood the act in its raw brutality. Looking at the boy and brooding over his story, I was overcome with seething anger and frustration. I felt nothing but unbridled loathing. He was the final insult, the ultimate gambit in a delicate human game. He had played the unspeakable trump card, leaving no chance for apology, discussion, or defense. It was the supreme act of selfish oneupmanship. Checkmate. The final buzzer. Game, set, and match.

I felt a deep pang of sympathy for the shattered girl, who for the rest of her life would remember how hair and brains had disintegrated on her doorstep. She would always see that crumpled body. I wondered if she would ever be the same. Could she start another relationship, no matter how casual and unattached? And, if so, could she maintain it? Would she be forever trapped by the arrogant self-destruction that found its way into her life? How could he do this to her? Or anyone? And what about his parents? How long and severe would be their innocent grief? I will never forget the sight of his half-towel head. That bastard. I would have slugged him but he was dead. There was nothing I could do. A half-smile was frozen on what remained of his face. And that is precisely how he planned it.

I had the same gut-level hatred for the woman with the bullet in her spine. Yet, as strong as these feelings were, I had to subordinate them and deal with her lab numbers and intravenous lines. The woman was still living and in all probability would continue to do so. She was, despite my opinion of her, a patient in need of treatment.

The surgeon arrived soon thereafter and the woman was whisked away. As I watched her bed roll down the hall, I wondered if she would some day regret that moment of revenge-filled passion. And, if so, would she grieve for its permanence? Would she long to run with her children or walk with her husband? Would she rage against her immobile sameness? Would she realize that self-infliction is almost always final? Would she know that she had taken half her life and parts of many others?

6.

With the critical woman gone I sent a nurse to prepare the long delayed leftover women for examination, then sorted through a few, quick mundane problems, the illnesses and afflictions that should have been seen during the day by a family doctor. I apologized to each person for the wait, which for some had been considerable, but reminded them that in the Emergency Room sometimes this is unavoidable. I kept one of these patients around for observation and further laboratory work.

Sandwiched amid the minor maladies was a child with cough and fever. The girl looked ill and repeatedly produced dark brown mucus from frequent paroxysms of bone-rattling cough. I listened to her chest and mentioned to her parents than an X-ray was in order. "It sounds like a pneumonia," I said.

Parents in general, even the more apprehensive ones, usually listen to my advice, perhaps ask a few questions, then go along with the stated plan. This child's parents took a somewhat different tack.

After I explained about the radiological procedure and what I expected to find, the father, a tall thin man wearing wire-rimmed glasses, a loud plaid shirt, and pants that stopped two inches above his shoe tops (a person no doubt resembling Washington Irving's conception of Ichabod Crane), stared intently at his severely dressed wife and said in a firm, much practiced voice, "Let's pray, Mother." Whereupon both of them dropped to their knees.

I was too surprised to speak. The man led off with an impassioned appeal for God to influence the X-ray film, then asked that this "malady" now afflicting his child's "tender and faithful lungs" be stricken, along with Satan, for good measure.

Coming from a staid Mormon background and not one

accustomed to such vocal and public displays of religious fervor, I was momentarily taken back and did not regain my composure for some minutes. By that time the kneeling man was finished and his wife had begun. I stood still and listened, uncertain whether to leave, stay, or kneel. I did not seem to be bothering them and, after all, it was my hospital, so I stayed and stood. Their voices carried loud and firm throughout the department. Every "Jesus" and "Lord" (pronounced "Lard"), of which there were many, rang off the walls and came shooting back. I noticed a man in the next bed reach over and pull back the curtain. He stuck his head around the corner with an extremely quizzical look on his face. I gestured slightly with my hand and he closed the drape.

As if this religious outburst had not been enough, the woman being readied for exam, the patient lady who had waited so long, began to shout also. Her exclamations were not, however, appeals to the deity, but cries of pain. Her voice had more volume than even the preacher's and carried through the air like a midsummer tornado, blasting everything in its path. The added commotion brought a second nurse running. And she seemed to do some good. In less than a minute she was down the hall and all was quiet again. I heard the suffering lady apologize and mention that she often got terrible gas pains but never quite as bad as that one. My attention was then returned to the impromptu worship service, where the wife had continued her impassioned appeal uninterrupted by the other woman's problem. Her husband, also undaunted, still nodded with each new thought and added an "amen" or "Hallelujah" where he deemed appropriate, a sort of Pentecostal punctuation. Then, as quickly as they had begun, they were finished. With a final "Praise the Lord," both stood and looked as if nothing unusual had happened, which I guess to them it hadn't. The father said that an X-ray would be fine and thanked me for my attention. All I could say was "You're welcome," turning my head slightly toward heaven as I did so.

Not wishing to experience another vocal typhoon, I hurried down to get that other woman checked before she screamed again. I briskly strode down the aisle, chart in hand,

and whipped open her cubicle curtain. Without looking at her, I stepped inside and whirled the curtain closed, then stepped to the edge of the bed. I found the woman's name on her chart and raised my face to greet her. It was all I could do to keep from gasping. It was all I could do to find the bedside, for in truth there was none. There was just person-side. I remembered then that the departing doctor had said this lady was fat but this understated the facts considerably. Obese was not word enough to describe such human tonnage. There might exist somewhere in a lexicographic text a more accurate and descriptive word for this mountain of flesh, but more likely it is still waiting to be invented.

A faded muumuu covered most of her substantial body acreage, draping like a huge flag over an abundant abdomen and thick, beefy thighs. Feet dangled from the end of this colossal person, no doubt glad for the brief breather. They looked like drowning sailors clinging to a ship. They were flat on the bottom, a visible proof of some physical law involving stress, mass, and structure.

I made my usual greeting and ask the woman what seemed to be bothering her. (I learned long ago not to begin by saying "What's the matter?" or "What's the problem?" for inevitably the answer comes back, "You're the doctor, you tell me." Each time I heard this I came nearer and nearer to a peptic ulcer. Still, that is not as bad as asking, "What brought you to the hospital?" to which the universal reply is, "My brother-in-law from Toledo" or "The bus." It took me some time to settle on "What's bothering you?" to which the only zinger is "Everything." I may get that ulcer after all.)

This woman did not say "everything." She told me in a clear and precise manner about waking to find blood on her sheets. She said that it might have been the beginning of her period but that her menses were so irregular, she wasn't sure. She said her cycles were messed up because of a "gland" condition.

I questioned the lady further as to the nature and character of the bleeding and attempted to pin down details regarding her day's progress. Then another pain wave hit. For me it was like standing in front of a lighthouse when the foghorn goes off. Tears formed in my eyes. I moved to the woman's side and made a futile effort at comfort by pressing her abdomen and saying that things would be all right. While this was going on, the curtain opened and a nurse poked in her head. I had not heard her footsteps. I had not heard anything but this agonized bellow for the past minute, and once it was past there was another minute of persistent buzzing in my ears.

I did a rapid physical assessment, more like a geographic survey than an examination, then said that a pelvic exam was in order. The woman consented. While instruments were being opened and the woman was being moved to the pelvic exam room, I attended to two minor, quiet problems. These done, I walked by Walter T.'s bed and found the space empty. He had been taken to the ICU. I smiled at my infected fourteen-year-old and wondered if the gynecologist had phoned back.

7.

The girl with the suspected pneumonia and the zealous parents was missing also. I imagined the man and wife mouthing some incantation over the X-ray machine. When I got to the nursing station, I sat down and trudged through the paperwork on all these people. Then I went to do that pelvic exam.

Medical instruments are made for a normal-sized population. Thus when abnormally large or small or unusually shaped people become ill, they face a problem. And so it was for my obese woman.

I entered the pelvic room and found her supine, with two elephantine feet pressing murderously on spindly, bowing metal stirrups. She had assumed what is poetically called the "lithotomy" position. I'm certain women have other names for it. The stirrups were set as far apart as possible, yet I could see only past midthigh. I knew we were in trouble. I summoned an extra nurse.

Then, like a baseball manager, I stationed my players. I put one nurse on either boulder-sized thigh and asked them to pull. There was a grunt from both pullers and a slight smacking sound as the two fleshy legs came further apart. I wedged in with both hands, but still found only leg. No vagina. Blindly I probed the hidden area with a silver speculum. Skin and fat quickly enveloped my Lilliputian appendage and its shiny instrument. With no end in reach, or sight, I quickly removed my hand lest I be pulled in further by some irresistible air pressure force. There was a smear of blood on the duckbilled metal speculum. I had not found her vaginal canal but had gotten close enough to verify that, indeed, the woman had been bleeding.

After a number of tries from a number of different angles, I finally gave up. And just in time too. No sooner had I set down my instrument and stood up than she had another pain spell. With the onset of cramps, her legs slammed shut like a castle door. Skin slapped against skin. It sounded like a rifle shot. Had I still been between them, I would have been crushed. I felt like the man who had just dived out the door before the bomb exploded. I stared back at those vice-grip thighs and wondered.

Fortunately, we were away from the main room, and this distance kept the noise somewhat confined. Although it concentrated the decibels for us inside, it kept any disturbance to other patients at a minimum.

This wave of spasms lasted longer than the last two. The sounds echoed and reverberated through the small room. The two nurses and I finally stepped away and casually covered our ears until the storm was over.

Reexamining the woman's stomach proved fruitless. It was like sticking my hand into soft sand. I buried my arm up to midwrist and still felt nothing but fat cells. Abdominal organs were hidden below, but, like an archeologist in search of Atlantis, I knew I would never find them.

Still the lady was sick. And still she needed a pelvic exam. I moved to plan B. I would ask the gynecologist to try. He had to see the fourteen-year-old girl anyway so, hopefully, he could zip over and examine the fat lady also. He must have dealt with obesity problems before and certainly had a reserve of trade secrets. I would be sure to have him check the child first, however. I did not want to incur his wrath any more than necessary.

In about five minutes after I got back to the nurses station, the unsuspecting doctor phoned and I explained both cases to him. I underexplained the fat part a bit. He agreed to come, and without comment. I appreciated that. There are some specialists who resent being called on holidays and weekends. But people get sick then and I need help. It is a pleasure when I don't have to beg.

Our Ob-Gyn man was small, not much larger than the fourteen-year-old. He had the chronically harried and tired look of someone who has stayed awake too many nights waiting for pregnant women to deliver. He arrived and removed his coat, purused both charts, and, at my urging, went in to look at the young girl first. With the large woman firmly ensconsed on the pelvic exam table, he chose to do the teenager's internal exam at the bedside. The curtain was closed and a portable light brought close, the same type of floor-standing circular lamp that other people use for reading. Below the curtain I saw a shaft of illumination and the doctor's feet. I heard the click of cold steel, then the girl's crying. It was over very quickly. The doctor stayed for a while and spoke to the child. His voice was quiet and indistinct; I could not make out the exact words. When he came back to the nursing station, his expression was unchanged. The exam light had been turned off and the wet instruments taken away.

"She will need a hysterectomy," the man said flatly, then sat down to jot a note on the chart.

"But she's only a child!" the twenty-one-year-old nurse blurted. The nurse who was fresh out of school training but was beginning to get her real training. "What about her future? What about children?" she asked, frustrated and angry. The young lady was badly shaken by this unexpected turn of events. She knew the girl was ill and had lied about her abortion but certainly she didn't need that kind of operation, not a hysterectomy. She must have felt ashamed and guilty, wishing she had never seen or touched the child. "How could we do this to her? How could she have done this to herself?" the young nurse said, turning first one way and then the other. It was then, for the first time, that she saw how other people's problems can stick to you and burn like napalm, or harden, like damp epoxy, unless you learn to dodge skillfully or wear a shield of indifference.

"She has a punctured uterus," the gynecologist said in answer to her questions, "and this has caused a significant infection to spread over all her pelvic cavity." His eyes did not deviate from his moving pen. His shield was up and in place. He could write behind it. "If she does not have immediate surgery," he continued, gaze down, "she will have no need for children because she will have no future. If I do not take out that decomposing womb, the girl will die." Then the doctor looked directly into the young nurse's eyes. His face was flat and hard like that of Byzantine icon.

I had to look very hard to see the quiver in the corner of his mouth and the tic in his right eyelid. He said no more. He did not want this to happen any more than we did. But it is difficult to operate when you are crying, so he remained calm. That's what shields are for.

I told him about the problem with the child's name and age and the whereabouts of her parents. (We discovered nothing, looking through her purse. We realized that fourteen year-olds simply don't have much to put in a wallet and have little need for identification. We found two folded one dollar bills and a torn magazine photo of John Travolta.)

The gynecologist then motioned to the young distressed nurse. She walked to his chair. He asked her, again without deviating his eyes from the paper upon which he was writing, if she would go back and speak to the child. "See if you can't get her to remember the name of her parents," the man said quietly. "This little lady is in for a very rocky time and she will need the comfort and support of her family." This was spoken with the sense of understanding that comes only from being a parent and having been called upon to give some measure of that same kind of understanding. I hoped that the family could give some, also. I hoped they could discover a reserve of compassion that would allow them to excuse their daughter for the disastrous decision she had made. I hoped they could overcome their own hurt and empathize instead of criticize. Their child was near death. She was facing surgery in which all her female parts were to be removed. I agreed that her future looked rocky and that she needed all the help she could get.

The operating room was engaged and the child made ready. Then the nurse returned with good news. After a crying session on both parts, the sick girl had given her correct name and phone number. She also confessed the name of her parents. Reality was sinking in.

The gynecologist called and spoke to the father directly. He did not give many details over the phone but impressed upon the man the urgency of his daughter's condition. He recommended that the family come immediately to the hospital. By the time the doctor had checked the porcine patient the parents had arrived.

My new nurse again headed to the lounge for a cigarette and cup of coffee. This time she puffed on the white burning stick with a vengeance, and took large, full gulps of steaming black liquid. Now she understood why nurse turnover in the Emergency Room is so high and why pills and alcohol seem a practical recourse.

The unflappable Gyn-man came back from his exam of the behemoth woman with a bemused smile on his face. He had, I discovered, devised a way to get at her vagina. With a folded sheet wrapped around each leg and a nurse pulling on each, the tree trunk thighs had been separated just long enough for the doctor to twirl his chair around and insert the backrest in the open space. This afforded him the extra push that was needed to complete the pelvic exam. Just before he left the room, he had been witness to one of her shouting jags, and for this I apologized. "That's quite all right," the other doctor said, "I expected as much." Then he picked up the phone and called his partner at home. The associate was asked to please come and assist. Yes, he knew it was Sunday night, but there were two cases that needed immediate attention and help was required. The partner said he would be right there.

"Transfer the large woman to Obstetrics right away," the visiting doctor directed our unit secretary, "and have them prepare for a delivery."

"A what?" I asked from across the room. I was holding another chart, a man with something in his eye, but quickly set it back in the rack.

"A delivery," the gynecologist repeated. "This woman is about to have a baby."

"You mean she's pregnant?"

"That's usually what precedes a delivery," the other doctor said without looking at me.

"But she never said that she was pregnant," I stated, befuddled and embarrassed that I had missed so obvious a condition.

"She didn't mention it," the doctor said, preparing to leave, "because she didn't know herself."

I had read about things like this, usually in the corner of the evening paper beneath some comical headline, or heard about it as the funny tag to a news broadcast, but I never imagined I would ever see one. The woman was so fat that she didn't know she was pregnant. And that wasn't even the most confusing aspect of the situation. I tried to imagine how she had gotten that way. I mean without the assistance of folded sheets and a chair.

"Boy, I'll bet she was surprised when you told her," I said chuckling.

"That's true," the consultant replied, striding to the door. "But no more surprised than her husband is going to be. I'm going out to break the news to him now." With that, he was gone. Never once during all of this did he show any emotion. Not one crack in his shield. He was a good and experienced doctor. But when he told the impending delivery story, a smile nearly came across his face.

I went back into the station and sat. I thought about the woman's water breaking and her going into labor. I thought about the sheets and the chair. I had to laugh. But that soon stopped. I heard the sudden jerking cry of another mother. The mother of the girl who was to have her pelvis cleaned out. The mother who had arrived with her husband while the fat lady was being examined. She too had just been told about the evening's events in the Emergency Room.

I watched the whimpering girl go by. She groaned in a thin child's voice, then vomited into a cardboard bucket. Her hair was matted with sweat. She looked like a baby. A worried, scared, hungry, tired baby. She looked too small to be that sick. For me the whole episode seemed so tragically remote, so divorced from reality. This girl should have been playing rock and roll records and talking on the phone. She should have been giggling and smiling at gangling boys. Going to the beach.

Dancing. Choosing Pepsi over Coke. She should have been doing those things like the rest of her friends. Instead of fighting for her life in a green, sterile operating room, where her child-bearing tissues would be removed. Instead of having her unborn family spilled into a metal basin, ripped out by steel forceps.

I needed a break. Once the child-woman was far enough down the hall to where I was certain not to pass her again, I excused myself and walked to the cafeteria. I thought perhaps eating something would calm my nerves and dull the image of that pathetic, festering child.

On the way I saw another ambulance pull up on the ramp. The red light was off; this meant it was nothing serious. The attendants moved about slowly. They leisurely assembled their rolling cart, then extricated a skeletal woman from the rear of their vehicle. As she went by, I noticed that a square of gauze was taped to her face.

I've been to Iowa. You might even say that I lived there for a while, on a pristine farm, in a tree-shaded house, surrounded by a well-groomed flower garden. If I lived there it was only for a night. That night at the hospital. In the cafeteria.

John sat while he talked, his body remaining rock still and his eyes glassed. He talked in a way most of us never will. He didn't speak of what he heard and saw now, but of what he had seen and heard then. He spoke with his mind's eye. From the heart.

His voice was low and calm, without a breath of excitement. Words clung to the air like dew on his beloved corn. For those few moments, he transcended both time and space.

The Iowa journey lasted but a short while for me. I was just a visitor. John was a resident. For him the trip was permanent. As the host, he allowed me in to see and hear, to feel and touch, to know his world. The world that he kept for himself and his wife. A world far removed from the pale green eating room in which we sat.

"The soil," he said, looking straight into my eyes, "that's what Iowa is all about, the soil." Then his gaze returned above my head. "No sir," he continued, "here you have dirt, Iowa has soil, acre after acre of rich black earth, just waiting— waiting for me and my corn." He leaned back in his chair. "That's what's in Iowa, the soil." He ran his right thumb across the tip of its four fingers. "Like cream," the grizzled old man began again, "it flows like cream across a plow. You could grow anything in that soil, pretty much anything."

John wore a wrinkled shirt with a frayed collar. His pants were marked with a gravy stain. A leather belt circled his trouser top but missed most of its loops. His shoes were dusty and unshined. No one lived with John. There was no one to comment upon his appearance or fix his sagging belt. He hadn't shaved in a day or two. A drawn face and tweed gray eyes only added to his somber mien.

Then he mentioned Mildred and everything changed. His voice suddenly sparkled like an opera tenor's, losing that tremulous waver common to old men. His eyes flashed with light. His skin glowed with color. He smiled.

Mildred, like so many of her generation, was born at home, in a house built by her father. "They don't put 'em up like that anymore," John said with a hand invisibly smoothing the stiff clapboard siding and carefully inset windows. He told of flowerbeds that hugged the structure in a loving grasp. And of dazzling white reflections in a noonday sun. And of the lazy looping willows.

Mildred grew up among undulating breadbasket hills, on land laden with corn. "Right near where I was raised," her husband stated proudly. "We lived but two farms down the road. I didn't know any other women." John shifted in his chair, "Mildred was the only girl for me. Had I looked," he said sincerely, "I couldn't have found one any better."

For a moment we sat in silence. Then he went on. "It wasn't like today. Now people marry someone from across the country, don't know a thing about their families. Not really," the old man said with a wise grin, "knowing anything about each other either."

John and Mildred dated five years before they were wed. There was no need to introduce families at the ceremony. Both vowed, that breezy spring day, to love, honor, and obey, through thick and thin. There had been a lot of thick. Now it was time for thin.

"Mildred never had to take an outside job," John said, leaning forward to emphasize the point. This lowered his line of vision to near my forehead. "Never worked outside the home," he repeated. "No sir, not even during the Depression." This was meant to be as much a compliment to himself as to the woman now lying in our E.R. bed. He was proud to have been able to provide during those lean years. He had seen his wife and family through hard times. And Mildred had always

148

worked in the home. Now there was no one for whom to provide, nor was there a home in which to work.

They were very proud of their children, John mentioned while stirring a cold cup of coffee with a bent spoon. The mug was full and had not given up a sip. He recounted their offspring by name and age, gave the name of each spouse and grandchild and everyone's whereabouts. This all took some time. But with John time was not important.

John talked about his spouse in loving and familiar terms. He called her "Mother" in the strange way older men sometimes refer to their wives. If she could have spoken, no doubt she would have called him "Dad."

The embodiment of an entire generation was contained in that man and his words. A generation raised to sacrifice, born to be parents. And they would continue to be so until their dying day. To them, parenthood was not something you did or did not choose, like a pair of shoes; it was something that you did, like eat and sleep. No one thought about it, or read magazine articles about it, or took classes in it. They just did it. And didn't ask questions. They were the parents we all want to have but don't want to be. They were parents even unto themselves.

During our conversation John used only plural pronouns and present-tense verbs, like "we are" or "she is." The words spoke of an eternal union, of a bond that was permanent, that would not be broken. I doubt if either person had ever said the word "divorce." He also spoke of a future. It would be hard to break this habit. Most likely he had done it all his life.

The room in which we sat was small and close, to me, confining and tense. But John never noticed. For him it was as wide as all Iowa and open as the wind over harvest grain. He did not smell the late night antisepsis or the day-old coffee. He was a farmer with his young bride. She was the girl in the gingham dress who laid pies to cool in the window.

I learned many things in the short time I spoke to that Iowa farmer. I learned all about life and the way things were. I learned from Mildred that night also. From her I learned about death and the way things are.

I know John had seen Mildred. Even though she lived in a nursing home, and had ever since her surgery, the staff said he visited often. He would, they said, sit quietly by her bedside and look out the window. Never speaking. He watched cars passing or clouds drifting by. On stormy days he followed the tracks of dying raindrops as they meandered toward the sill. When an hour was past, he quietly slipped out. All the while Mildred lay still as stone. Immobile. Breathing slowly through the gauze. John came three times a week, like clockwork.

The woman, pale and limp, shrouded in a shabby blue blanket, was wheeled through the Emergency Room door. Without stopping at the desk, her attendants rolled her directly to a bed. It took only one person to lift and carry her across. The empty gurney made a slight chirping noise, like the sound of excited birds, as it traveled back up the hall and was reloaded in the ambulance.

John had come in behind. I caught both of them at the door. He did not say good-bye to his wife nor make any motion to her whatever. He walked directly to the cafeteria. He knew where it was; he had been there before.

Just as I got back to the department, I received a call from Mildred's doctor. He wanted to alert us to her arrival. He said that he didn't think there was anything left to do for the woman and to let her pass quietly. The nursing home did not want her to die there—something about paperwork, he said. Despite the hour, her doctor's voice was calm and resolute but laced with a sad tone that made me take notice. It was a voice that understood. Then he warned me about her face.

Death arrives in many ways. For a fortunate few it comes quickly, with a car crash or plane wreck, perhaps a sudden heart attack. Others pass in their sleep and, except for a muffled moan or a quick leg jerk, they die unnoticed. A bedmate will awake to find his partner gone. And wonder why he wasn't disturbed.

These are the lucky ones, the blessed few, because for

some, like John and Mildred, death is known and expected. It becomes a constant companion, a third spouse, someone who comes to be known intimately, every line and wrinkle, every motion and odor. The waiters come to know death, eventually better even than they know themselves.

In the beginning, I'm sure, those who know of Death must dismiss his presence. In the beginning he is only words and numbers, letters printed on a sheet or a nervous look upon a doctor's face. But as the lumps grow and the pain increases, his icy fingers become reality, like the image of a surfacing diver slowly taking shape. Until at last, he is there to stay. After Mildred's operation, death came to stay.

It must be very difficult to expand to three a relationship that has for fifty years been just two. To wedge another party between man and wife, like a jealous lover who soon demands first attention and gets it. It must be difficult to face an interloper to whom emotional homage must be paid. For the companion Death, once he has arrived, does not leave.

To the religious person, death in the beginning takes on a different complexion. Some claim it is just another step in a long journey, a portal through which they must pass, an ordeal before the reward. For a while they handle it best. Yet they too one day must face the companion face to face. Alone. Nose to nose.

I admire those who know and admit to being frightened. Those who grimace at the thought and recoil from the day. It is a much simpler and cleaner approach. They keep the jack-in-the-box open and study the clown. He does not burst past their face and cause them to scream. When the time comes, they simply stand up and are knocked down.

John faced his wife's illness in a forgetting way. He chose to hide. Death was in the desert, not on the farm. So he traveled to Iowa, back to the farm. Again he ate window-cooled pies and tilled brown, giving soil. Mildred was a shadow on the shade, seen from a far field, moving easily about the house.

No one knew how Mildred faced death. She couldn't talk. Nor had she the strength to write. I spoke to her as she lay on our thin metal bed but I don't know if she understood.

Mildred had cancer. It started with a lump in her nose, which she chose to ignore. To her it was not cancer until a doctor told her it was cancer. So she kept the lump and avoided the doctor. When another bump appeared inside her mouth; even she could dismiss things no longer. A biopsy was taken. It proved malignant.

Her doctor said Mildred originally declined surgery but, at the urging of her husband, she was finally convinced to go ahead. Perhaps they didn't fully understand the implications. After the operation, neither John nor Mildred was ever the same.

It was that surgery, the operation he pushed for his wife to have, that, as much as anything, drove John back to Iowa. After the operation he looked at Mildred only once. Then he left for the farm.

There are certain things in human life, and medicine in particular, that are beyond comment or judgment. They are neither right nor wrong: They just are. Cancer is one of them. Why does it exist? I don't know. There is no answer. There is cancer because there is cancer. Just as there are trees because there are trees. No reason.

To understand the therapy for cancer, one has to adopt a similar approach. There is a problem and a solution. Although often heart-rending and bizarre, the solutions are just that— solutions. And so it was with Mildred.

Mildred wore a large piece of gauze taped to her face. The cloth began just below her eyes and extended down to nearly cover her chin. The sides went close to each ear. There was no bulge in the middle. For reasons which I can never explain, I lifted that piece of gauze.

Where a nose and mouth should have been there was nothing. Just a hole. A large, gaping cavern. No lips. No nose. No cheeks. No nothing. And the cavity was deep, as if scooped out by a small shovel. This was, I imagined, not too far from the surgical truth.

The hole was not, however, empty.

It was full of live maggots.

Full of maggots, not because of neglectful care but because they had been placed there. The carnivorous insects eat dead tissue, and Mildred's face was dead tissue. They kept her wound clean. A wound which would never heal. This is what I mean by a solution. A result. A result that is just there, like the trees. There was nothing to say.

I pictured John, that day after surgery, doing the same thing I had done, lifting the gauze. I imagined him staring for a moment, retaping the cotton cloth, then leaving for Iowa. Forever.

I replaced the mask, once again covering that swarming facial mass, then grasped both bedrails for support. They rattled a soft, metallic tune. Had I looked any longer, I would have vomited. Or left for somewhere myself.

Since that night I have thought about many things, among them, death, illness, treatment, dying, and my relationship to each. I have thought long and hard but still have no answers. I always end up back with the trees.

I left John in the cafeteria, where he stayed until they took Mildred away. He followed her out to the hearse and watched the limousine drive away. Then he walked home.

It was a good many minutes before I could see any other patients, and there were a number that needed seeing. It was even longer before I could purge the image of Mildred's face from my mind. Sometimes I wish I had never lifted that piece of gauze. It made me think over my life and what things are really all about. It made me realize the egotistical futility of self-pity. No matter what my problems were, someone's burden was always worse. And all because I lifted that piece of gauze. But, after all, her doctor had warned me.

9.

In the E.R. it's funny how things run in streaks, as if obeying some natural law of illness. Patients with similar complaints seem to accumulate at certain times, or all patients one day will be around the same age. I have had periods in which everyone seemed to do well and periods when everyone did poorly. That Sunday night served up a double dose of coincidence; most of the patients seemed to be children. And most of them were very sick.

After Mildred was removed, things were quiet for a while. Nurses made the beds, turning out fresh sheets, replacing the smudged bloody ones. Skinny, black mattresses were scrubbed shiny. The Emergency Room was empty, catching its breath, waiting for the next wave of attackers. To look down the sentinel row of unoccupied beds and then to stare up an empty hall is a feeling similar, no doubt, to being in a hurricane's eye. You have just been through rough weather and you know it will be rough again very soon, but for now things are serene and eminently calm. There is no one crying and no one running. But outside the winds are circling.

I wandered into the nurses' lounge and opened a can of soda. A television was playing from an elevated shelf but no one took any notice. The picture flickered but the sound was off. I thumbed through an old newspaper taken from a pile scattered on the floor, glanced briefly at the headlines, then concentrated on the sports page. One by one the nurses filed in and poured themselves a cup of coffee. The aluminum brewer was hot and steaming. It stayed on twenty-four hours a day. If there were to be a shift without coffee, the staff would get very agitated.

Quickly all the seats were filled. Conversation spread in every direction.

"Doctor Seager, you know that you missed Helen's send off party last week?"

"Was that last week?"

"I sent you an invitation for Friday the nineteenth."

"Was last Friday the nineteenth already?"

"Yes it was."

"I'll be darned," I said, checking the date on my newspaper. "My calendar must have stopped."

Since I began working in the Emergency Room, I have developed the ability to forget, or perhaps, better stated, the inability to remember, past events and patients. I know my subconscious does this on purpose, as protection. Like a knight in Freudian armor, it guards me from memories that would haunt and cripple me, should they be allowed free reign. But this can be a problem also. Often another doctor will stop by and ask me about a recent patient. Even if he gives me the name, the time that I saw him, and what was wrong, I have to sift my mental nooks diligently to recall anything at all about the case. This can be very embarrassing. But, as I said, it's subconscious and beyond my control. Last year I was subpoenaed to testify regarding an assault case. Supposedly, I had treated the victim after his attack, at least the chart said that I had. No doubt the prosecution had counted on me to give a detailed description of the plaintiff's wounds and the service we rendered. And I would have liked to have done this. But I couldn't. The time between attack and trial was a year and one half and by then my subconscious had carried the memory very far away. I could not remember a thing. Not the man. Or his injury. Or his care. Nothing. Even with the old chart in hand I could not summon one shred of fact. I recognized my writing but felt as if I were looking at some foreign script. Still I did as the court requested and appeared at the specified time. Perhaps, I thought, if I could see the victim's face, my memory would be jogged. But it wasn't. The courtroom was filled with total strangers, each face new, none of which brought a glimmer of recognition.

156

Then I spotted someone whom I thought might be the victim. I studied his face very carefully and had even convinced myself that I could restructure the incident, putting him on the chart on the night in question. When the trial was called to order I discovered the man to be the defendant, the man who had done the beating. That's when I talked to the attorney for the county. He looked dejected and angry but was forced to excuse me. He ripped a sheet from an elongated yellow pad and wadded it with disgust.

I say this because it was not until well into Sunday evening, after the television stations had melted into a maze of frantic static, that I thought about the two men who had been operated upon the night before. In a burst of painful recall, the blood decision and all its agony came back to me. I realized that I had no idea how either patient was doing, indeed whether they were still alive. I laid my paper aside, took a final gulp from a soda can, and excused myself.

Certainly, I concluded, both men were still in Intensive Care, so I told the nurses I was headed there and walked down the hall toward the elevators. I pushed the "Up" button and leaned against the wall. A small light above my head lit the number "Six" and an arrow pointed down. The hospital was tormentingly quiet. I even heard clicks as the elevator lights went on in descending order, 6, 5, 4, 3 . . . then I heard the hospital doors slide open. The noise of a million raindrops pelting the pavement and the swoosh of a passing car instantly invaded my silence. Two big electric doors cruised easily on their metal runners as feet pounded into the cavernous hallway. It is quite normal for people to run through the emergency entrance. It was unusual, however, to hear frantic steps coming from the front door.

Announcing itself with a loud ding, my elevator arrived. I paid no attention but stepped into the hall instead. Just inside the gaping glass doors, outlined by vertical rainsheets, was a man carrying a little girl. He was pacing one direction and then the next, obviously confused and looking for help. A janitor appeared and directed him to the Emergency Room. Man and child were by me in a flash, passing so close that I could feel hot breath. Close behind, having herself just burst through the still-open door, was the child's mother. She went by in equal haste. I forgot about my elevator trip.

I could easily follow the family's trail: there was blood dripping on the floor. Small, evenly spaced blobs of red led directly to the first E.R. bed. There I found the child. One nurse was already assembling suction equipment while another roped the terror-stricken parents with her open arms, herding them out to the front desk. For now they would only be in the way. Many parents faint during scenes like this. We needed only one patient.

I entered the treatment area through a side door, thus avoiding an immediate confrontation with the anguished family. We would have time to talk later. At the bedside, the first nurse had completed her vacuum assembly and was jamming a hose between the child's chalk-milk teeth. The small mouth fell open easily, letting the plastic tip slide in. Bright crimson blood quickly filled the extracting line and collected in a plastic wall bottle.

The child was waxen and limp, the color of leeched protoplasm. The color of young life nearly lost. I touched her cool hands, they were immobile. I put a wooden tongue depresser into her scarlet stained mouth. Again, she offered no resistance. That was a bad sign. In general, only when children are gravely ill will they allow such manipulation. Her arms hung like paper banners. A second nurse had to hold the girl's head straight.

A third nurse had opened a bottle of intravenous solution and was probing for a flaccid vein. When her needle punctured the skin, the child didn't flinch.

"Tell me the story," I said, stepping to a spot directly in front of the girl.

"The child had her tonsils out three days ago," the mouth-cleaning nurse said, amid the sump and suck noise that her vacuum created, "and about fifteen minutes ago everything let loose. She must have popped her stitches. If we don't stop this bleeding," the woman said, momentarily removing her

158

plastic pipe and manually wiping a large clot from the tip, "this child is going to die. She is going to bleed to death."

And the nurse was right. For just then the girl sat straight and vomited. Only it wasn't vomit that came out, it was blood. Burgundy liquid splattered over the child's clothing, over the nurse, and over me. I estimated she had evacuated at least half a unit of heme from her stomach, about one-sixth of her total circulation volume. And she was still swallowing. Soon that one-sixth would be one half, and then all.

A hemorrhaging throat is a difficult place to attack. The tissue is fleshy, vascular, and hard to handle. Also, it is in an enclosed, distant location, the same location through which the patient must also breathe. It can become a nightmare.

There are days in the Emergency Room, indeed entire weeks, when I feel that nothing of any import has been accomplished. All the sore throats and colds will get better no matter what we do. Most anyone can learn to splint a foot or suture a laceration. And all the code arrests die. Then something will occur that makes the drudge worthwhile. Something that erases the memory of a thousand dull cases and a hundred losing battles with death. Occasionally we will do something heroic. Something that literally snatches life back from death, something of which we can be proud. One of those things happened with that little girl.

In the next minute we saved her life.

As I said, bleeding in the throat is difficult to control, mainly because pressure is hard to apply. First I tried my hands but found that her mouth was too small. Next came a cloth tied to the end of a plastic tube. I pushed the rag in but quickly had to release it. She was gasping for air. And still the sucking and blood swallowing continued. I grabbed a handful of Q-tips but they proved unwieldy. I couldn't hold enough to do any good. It was like eating with twenty chopsticks. I tossed the tangled swabs to the floor. I was sweating, cold and angry. I slammed my fist into the bed mattress. The child didn't notice. Her throat was now visibly bulging with each swallow of blood. Soon she would vomit again. I turned away to think and inadvertently

159

looked into the hallway. There my eye was caught by a vaginal inspection tray, the one left by the Ob-Gyn doctor. The tray was just outside our small pelvic room, waiting to be resterilized. For some reason, amid a tangle of soiled instruments and matted wet gauze, bunched below two wadded green towels, I saw two sticks. They were the wooden ends of large vaginal tampons, giant cotton swabs-on-a-stick. They are used to stanch bleeding high up in the vaginal canal. The similarity between that and my situation suddenly struck me. I dashed over and picked up the unused drumsticks. In my haste I knocked the tray over, spilling speculums and cloth all over the floor. Sticks in hand, I was back at the bedside.

Quickly their paper coverings were torn off. Then, like a picador at the bullring, I clutched them in my fists and plunged those billowy tufts into the child's open mouth. I pushed down and out as hard as I could. One white pledget was held against each spouting tonsil bed.

For better traction I jumped on the bed and straddled the child with my knees. The nurse let out an involuntary gasp. And then we waited. In thirty seconds the suction began to clear. The sound of air became more prominent because the scavenging tip was no longer finding blood. Sprung vessels had clamped closed.

By then the intravenous line was wide and flowing, replacing lost fluid volume. Later the girl would require transfusion but right now she needed something to pump in her veins and saline would do just fine. She opened her eyes and smiled around the sticks in her mouth. I smiled back. One of the nurses cried.

I knelt on the bed for what seemed an eternity. Then, with anxious trepidation, I let loose one of the fiber batons. Slowly the soggy instrument was extricated. There was no bleeding underneath. I let the other go. Again nothing. Her throat was dry. To be sure it stayed that way, I swabbed the dangerous areas with silver nitrate, a chemical cautery, the same thing used to control nosebleeds. It scorched that friable tender tissue into a tough, coagulated scab. The worst was over.

160

Soon laboratory blood was flowing instead of saline, and our ear, nose, and throat doctor was on the way. The child was speaking and even laughed. Her parents were ebullient. They gestured with wide motions and talked animatedly. Their joy was that of those who know the sting of true horror. They had lost their child and reclaimed her again. Now that child's every word and action, previously taken for granted, was a source of pride and wonder. Their lives and relationship would never be the same.

10.

My wife is fond of saying that there exists a balance and harmony in life. And I think she is right in the sense that things do tend to even out over the long run. Good will return good—that's the harmony part—and for every serendipity there will be a corresponding misfortune—that's the balance part. For every tragic encounter there will be a funny one. And for every life that may be saved, there may be a life lost.

Years may pass between connecting links. Often I have to think carefully to remember a remote mirror event. In this particular case, the girl spared from the bleeding throat, I had to wait only a few seconds to see whether or not nature would exert an actuarial balance and restore perfect-pitch harmony. I had saved a child. The books were unbalanced. Was an account open? Would I now lose a child? No sooner had I delivered the living child to her ecstatic parents than two shrill beeps reverberated through the Emergency Room. All motion ceased and we exchanged glances. It was the paramedics again. The parents attending to their living child took no notice. Somewhere in town, on the other end of that shortwave line, parents were attending another child.

"This is Life Rescue," said a static-filled voice. I picked up the land-line receiver.

"This is Doctor Seager. Go ahead, please."

"Doctor, this is paramedic Jones. We are at the scene of a pediatric drowning. The child was submerged for approximately five minutes prior to our arrival. There was no resuscitation effort in progress...

And so it began. The balance part.

In our town it is the swimming pool. Other cities lose their children to accidents, poison, beatings, but here, although we have similar tragedies, it's swimming pools. And the stories are always the same. "I was just gone for a minute," the parents say, "...to answer the door...to talk on the phone...to this or that...." Even though it was late, I knew I would hear the same story tonight. "I just left him for a minute to...."

While the nurses readied the code room, I waited. I took a drink of water, scooping ice from the hallway machine, slowly filling my cup. I wasn't nervous, nor was the staff. We had done this all before and we would undoubtedly do it again. So we just got prepared and waited.

In all too short a time the mechanical doors flew open. Scarlet flashing lights again flickered through the moving translucent glass, bursting to vivid red as the outside rushed in. Two blue-suited firemen were running alongside a careening cart. One held aloft a bottle of intravenous fluid. The other pushed on a small chest, rapidly, using only three fingers. An ambulance driver followed the pair squeezing a black bag connected to a very thin plastic hose that disappeared down a very small throat.

In a blur, the child was off the gurney and onto the code room bed. He was now mine. If this little person were to live, I thought then, if he were ever to have school, friends, a wedding, ball games, fights, races, Christmas, children, a job, old age, tomorrow, anything, he had to survive the next thirty minutes.

I rushed to his bedside and looked down. And then it hit, as it does everytime I do this. I got that same familiar feeling. How long the feeling lasted, I can't tell. A moment? A minute? An hour? I don't know. But suddenly there was no noise. No rushing nurses or heated discussion. No medicine or I.V. lines. Suddenly there was just me and that boy. That boy lying so peacefully on the cart. That boy with his loving face caught as if in a picture frame. That tiny boy waiting obediently to die.

In my mind I have a gallery of these pictures, a score or more, collected over a number of years. These same face-pictures are in many parents' minds also. They are stored like books that only we share. But their books are closed. My album keeps on growing, year after year, face after face. And it will continue to grow, I guess, until the sheer weight and number allow me to forget.

I reached out and touched his cheek. It was smooth and soft, as are those of other children. It was also very wet and cold, not like those of other children.

The early minutes were easy. We followed a preset protocol. The child was probed and analyzed, plugged into our monitors; he had his body fluids extracted for laboratory examination. In the past this path had led to some success. We hoped for the best.

Tempers and tensions, already strained, were running high. Elbows bumped and bodies collided. Too many people were trying to encircle too small an area. Sometimes my orders were not heard above the bustle and they had to be repeated. But that didn't matter. Everyone was doing all he could.

Although my speaking was directed at the other people, my thoughts were not. My thoughts were directed at the child.

"Breathe, little boy, breathe."

"Beat, little heart, beat."

With every new drug or body-piercing procedure, I thought the same thing.

"Breathe, little boy, breathe."

"Beat, little heart, beat."

I said it over and over. But it was doing no good.

After many futile minutes, I needed a break. For just a while, I needed time to think and assess. I needed water.

Stepping into the hallway, I turned to the fountain. At first I thought the corridor was empty, just rows of doors standing erect above geometric lines of linoleum, the pattern, like two mirrors placed face to face, repeating into infinity. Then I saw him. One doorway wasn't empty. It contained a man. I could see his head and shoulders angled into the hall. He was looking at me.

Even from a distance I could see him trembling. They were fine rapid oscillations, but I could see them nonetheless. His face was white, the color of snow on a mountain slope. His eyes were wide with pupils dilated. He looked like the jackrabbits that you see at night in the Nevada desert. The ones that are hypnotized by your oncoming headlights. Jackrabbits that leap gracefully into the air just before they are crushed by your car.

It was probably a coincidence that I had walked into the hallway at the same time he had chosen to look out. But I'm not sure. He may have been looking down the hall all this time.

I knew who he was, the other man in the hallway, the man with the full moon eyes. I had seen his face before, only in miniature. I had seen those same features staring up from a bed, reflecting ceiling lights from a cyanotic surface. I had seen the same sandy hair and the same small nose. He was the boy's father.

I turned away quickly, pretending not to notice. Perhaps he doesn't know who I am, I thought. But that was not the case. I could tell by the way he stared, desperate for a sign of hope, a smile, a wave, a nod, anything. But I had no hope to give. I simply could not face the situation, so I spun away. I could not crush that man like a jackrabbit. I could not take his son away. At least not yet.

At the fountain I was no longer thirsty. My mouth was tacky, like gum left on the hot pavement, my throat was too tight to swallow. I wished only that I could dive into that arching clear, crystal water stream and float down the drain.

I stood at the cooler for a good long time letting its cool liquid bathe my lips. I stood and I listened. I could not see the others but I could hear them. The man in the room at the other end of the hall was not alone. There were other men and women with him and they were all crying. From this symphony of voices I focused on one. Like the melancholy cry of a solitary bird over a still lake, one sound rose above the rest. It was a mother's wail. It was the grief of a woman who had brought a life into the world, a life that now, it seemed, I would usher out.

A few fast steps and I was back to the code room. Inside, things were essentially the same except that the boy had had his soggy clothing removed and was now partially covered by a white sheet. His bare chest, which had for the past half hour been artificially compressed, like an accordion, began, with each new external push, to crack softly. The continual force required to extract blood from the youth's inert heart had broken his ribs.

As do most dying hearts, this boy's ventricles were fibrillating. In an effort to establish itself again in the world, his heart was contracting crazily. The only cure for this is, in essence, cardiac electrocution. Large doses of electricity would have to be sent directly through the child's thorax.

This was done twice. But the heart did not respond. Sometimes after such a shock, a heart will return to it's natural rhythm. This boy's did not.

Regardless of the heart's electrical outcome, the skin always suffers from such an action. A huge, seering charge invariably leaves rings where the driving paddles rested on the surface. This boy had two sets.

Numerous drugs had by now also been given, forced through plastic tubes in his arm or jabbed directly into his frantic heart. He had been given drugs to stimulate his heart contractions and drugs to combat acid accumulation in his bloodstream, drugs to correct chemical abnormalities in his serum and drugs to stop a mid-effort seizure. Drugs used in wisdom, hope, and desperation. And still there was nothing.

Medicine as portrayed on television is a clean, precise science. The prototype physician makes a lifesaving gesture, straightens his tie, and exits quietly. Cut to commercial. In reality things are very different. And very messy. In reality, the fight for life is sticky and it smells. Everything and everybody ends up covered with blood, urine, or vomit. The human body rarely gives up the ghost angelically, but instead literally oozes and expels itself to death. A soul exits in viscous, vile secretions, pushing the essence of existence through relaxed alimentary openings.

This boy vomited also. Amber acrid slime erupted like a volcano and gloved the hands of those working his breathing bag. It convulsed from his mouth and tumbled like putrid lava down both cheeks, puddling on the sheet. A suction hose quickly evacuated his tiny mouth.

And blood was everywhere. Not the poetic flowing liquid of detective novels but the congealed real kind. Corpuscles were scattered about like tiny dots in a pointillistic painting. The fluid spattered my glasses. I could taste the dry drops that dotted my lips.

It is difficult to imagine the horror this frantic ensemble creates. Or the lonely frustrating anger. Most people scarcely know it exists. When they think of swimming pools they think of water polo and swimming races, of suntan oil and iced tea. They don't think of vomit and blood. They think of pleasant poolside chatter under a warm, browning sun. They don't think of their child stumbling in during the night. They don't think of tile walls and the antiseptic smell. Or the words, "Your son is dead."

And this one was dead. Nothing we had done so far seemed to help and nothing more that we were to do did either. His wildly contracting heart slowly turned into a listless still one. His skin turned a final dusky shade that said there would be no reversal. A thin mucous glaze formed over both eyes. As I stood back and nodded, thus halting the resuscitation effort, I thought of the other children I had seen like this. I thought how much they looked like they were only sleeping. Old people die; children sleep. Isn't that the way it is supposed to be? "Just resting, Sir, I'll be up in a minute." If those words came from that tiny lifeless body, no one would have been surprised. But only because we wanted so very much for it to be that way.

It now fell upon me to tell the parents, the wailing mother and wild-eyed father, that things had come to an end. When I entered that small hall's-end room, they were both on the edge of the sofa. Others were with them but they sat back, somewhat more relaxed. I said I was sorry but their child was dead. The mother screamed, her sorrow bursting outward. The father twitched and jerked straight back, like an electric current had been run through the couch. He turned his anguish inward. I said again how sorry I was and then excused myself, leaving the grieving group in the hands of an experienced nurse and a hastily called social worker. I remember someone telling me later that the child had wandered out through an open door while the parents were entertaining friends. They thought that he was in bed. It was, after all, very late at night.

I bit my lip all the way back to my office, passing a number of unseen patients and their blank charts. My head was aimed directly forward. I struggled to see through wet and blurring eyes.

Once alone, I sat on a stark unmade bed and fought back the tears. I held firmly to the edge, determined not to cry. I had long ago sworn not to let the horror and inequity of life overcome me. I had sworn to be above senseless tragedy and its web of sorrow, but this time I had to resort to mental games and reasoned theologic syllogisms to remain so. If there truly were a God, I thought, then this all must have some purpose, it must someday mean something. It must be credited to an eternal suffering account, somehow making us better people. And if deity wasn't? Then whether a kid fell into a swimming pool or not really didn't matter after all. This approach worked for a while but eventually eroded, and I could think of no other explanation. So, like the nurses before me, I cried.

At first the tears were small and concentrated, squeezed out through rusty ducts atrophied from disuse. But each succeeding drop came more easily. Soon the track was greased and the tears were flowing freely. At last winding rivulets twisted down my cheeks and dripped from my chin. They were tears for that little boy, tears for his parents, tears for all parents. I licked the salty stream, then buried my face in a pillow so no one would hear. So no one would know that I was crying and had broken my vow.

After some minutes I stood and made for the bathroom sink. I washed my face without looking in the mirror. Then I went back to the nursing station. I had other people to treat and other problems to solve. On the way I passed a small mortuary bag that lay folded on a cart.

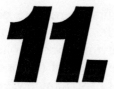

11.

The child with the infected chest and the evangelic parents had returned from Radiology. I hoped that her pneumonia would be small and easily treated. I also hoped the mother and father would accept an antibiotic prescription without too much fanfare. I was in no mood for a camp revival prayer over my pad and pen.

An orderly handed me the child's film, and I flipped it to a view box. From a distance I scanned her dome-shaped lungs; they looked like two side-by-side haystacks, each with one flat side. The actual breathing organs were dark where a radiation beam had penetrated normal tissue and white where electrons had met bone or disease. Amid a ghostly picket fence of ribs was a baseball-sized chunk of pneumonia. The light box was turned off and the X-ray taken down. Then I sat to write the antidote prescription. I had written the girl's name and the words "ampicillin 250 mg" when the lights went out.

With a fatal B-movie type groan, the airconditioner fans spun to a stop. The hall lights dimmed, then winked black. One small red emergency bulb, hung above a distant back doorway for just this emergency, struck up—keeping the Emergency Room from total darkness. Instead of a pitch-black coffin we were now in a huge photo lab. Then for a brief hope-charged moment the lights wavered and the fans sighed, but both died once more. I knew we had a backup power system and I suspected that it too had failed, because this time even the little red light went out.

The darkness, like a child, took time to blossom and mature. In a minute or so my eyes had lost all memory of light. Like fire under water, my retinal rods and cones had shut down. After grasping for any shred of illumination, my optic nerve quieted like a dead snake. The settling darkness brought a respectful silence, almost cathedral-like. At first there were occasional shouts into the ink. "What happened?" "Hey!" "What the . . .?" But these quickly stopped. Then everything was absolutely still. And we remained this way until the father of the pneumonia-infected child spoke again. "Jesus Christ Almighty," the man said in a reverential tone. For the first time he seemed appropriate.

A nurse and I made our way to the hallway, where, with one palm held close against the side wall, we reached the swinging doors. Our steps in the ebony corridor bounced and caromed like rocks thrown down a deep well.

In the actual waiting room there was a bit of light. From a single power pole stationed across the road, one emergency street lamp cast a slight gray haze that filtered limply in through the front glass doors. Outlined against this wool-gray background the persons in the sitting room looked like faceless apparitions. Every so often one of these amorphous zombies would rise and bend over the drinking fountain. Although the room contained at least ten people, there was not a single word being exchanged. It was the first time I could remember seeing the waiting area without the television going.

"Name, please," I heard from behind me, back at the sign-in station. It was the voice of our front reception clerk. I turned and saw a shaft of light aimed over her typing fingers. There was suddenly a faint chatter in the air. Seated in front of the woman was a man offering some complaint. Behind her was a security guard shining a flashlight over each shoulder. "Address" she said, continuing, "You're something else," I remarked to the industrious woman. And I meant it.

Back through the doors and it was once again dark. That is until I saw the bright darting shafts. From the nursing station there now came intermittent bursts of light like lightning over a black lake. The staff were scurrying about their business, each with a flashlight in his or her hands. They looked like huge fireflies or miners emerging from a mountain.

"Hello," I said, leaning in the station door. "Did you know that the lights were out?" "Very funny," the charge nurse replied, her voice coming from behind one of the beams. "Come in, we need your help to pass out lights." Before I could answer, an armful of drugstore flashlights was handed to me. Then a hand from an unseen body pulled me into the patient area, where I began distributing my wares.

At the end of the line was a man with a sprained ankle. I told him that we would get him down to X-ray as soon as our power problem was straightened out. Turning on his light, he said he understood, that the lights were out at his house too but that he had come to the E.R. anyway because he couldn't imagine the hospital would be hooked to the same electrical source, one that could go out so easily, and if they were hooked to the same power supply, then certainly they would have a backup system that worked, an emergency generator or something—you know, like for someone who was in surgery or on a breathing machine at the time, so that's why he came, he said, but once he saw that our building was dark also he thought he might as well come in and wait, seeing as how he had come this far already and that it was dark at his house too. He could wait for the lights here as well as there, he said. I said that I understood. Which of course I didn't. I couldn't figure out why a hospital would have a power system that could so easily be stricken down either. And there very well might have been someone in surgery. I didn't tell the sprained ankle man any of that, I let it go with, "I understand."

Without further words one of the beams approached and a hand again took my arm. This time I was guided toward the code room as the nurse shone her light ahead. Before us, familiar objects took on an ominous cast. Stools and chairs leapt in and out of the hand-held light. Involuntarily, I took short, halting steps, afraid that at any instant I would bark my shins.

Inside, the special room looked like a Druidic seance. A bright circle of faces was gathered around a prone, dark form. It was the regular trauma team and their flashlights. Each person was attending to his or her job in the darkness. Mostly, they were cursing the situation and jerking around their beams. Bodies collided. A light dropped. "Shit!" someone said. "Ouch!" another shouted as he banged his head on the table while reaching down for the fallen flash. Someone nudged me closer to this medical coven.

Spotting the blue shirt of a fire department paramedic, I made my way to him. "What happened?" I asked. He jumped and looked around. I reached over to the counter, picked up a stray light, and shone it up to my face, like some spookhouse trick. "It's me . . . Dr. Seager," I said with what must have been a very ghoulish grin. "What happened?"

The man on the table, he explained to me, had skidded in his car and slammed into a telephone pole. Then the medic gave me the approximate speed at impact, advised me of the man's vital signs at the scene, and told me that the fellow's breathing had worsened somewhat during the trip in.

With this done, he packed to leave. At the door he turned and said, "We bring a patient into this black funhouse and you ask me 'what happened?' " I thought he was joking and laughed, but then I wasn't sure because he had put his light away and I couldn't see his face.

When the patient groaned, I turned back to see my Druids still at work, probing, measuring, writing, as a dark puddle formed on the floor. Blood was dripping from an outstretched arm, an arm perforated by a thousand needle sticks. "I give up!" shouted a voice in the dark; then someone threw down an I.V. needle and tubing. It disappeared from the footlights. "Let me try," another voice said, and another needle hole was punched in the runny arm. Finally, hole one thousand and twenty struck blood and soon water was running into the perforated appendage. The lab had equal difficulty. It is hard enough to draw blood from a well-lit arm, never mind one in the dark with a dozen people crowding around. The lab girl drilled feverishly. And in due time enough tubes were filled with blood. The woman heaved a relieved sigh and stepped out of the proscenium.

Taking X-rays was no easier. With great effort a lumbering portable radiation machine was clumsily driven into the small room. It's grumbling motor stopped when the huge iron body was pressed against the thin small bed and an attached metal head was poised over the patient's shadowy abdomen. "Everyone out," an anonymous voice shouted. The rays were going to be loosed. In seconds, the entire staff had stumbled into the nursing station proper while the enormous machine clicked softly as its handler directed, "Breathe deeply and hold it." The man made a quick burst in for a change of film and took another shot. Then the huge glowering lizard retraced its steps and faded down the hall.

I checked the I.V. line; drops were percolating at a good steady rate. A Foley catheter had somehow been inserted in the man's urethra and was tapping yellow urine from his bladder. Considering the size of the penile meatus and the prohibitive conditions, this technical feat deserved mention. "Did this guy come in with a Foley?" I asked the crowd. "No, sir, I put it in," someone replied from the back. "Thank you, whoever you are," I said with genuine admiration.

The staff then gathered around the man and beamed their lights as one. With this I was able to get a fairly good view of the fellow and do a reasonable physical exam. His head appeared to be intact; he even moaned when I called to him. No doubt the man would rouse from this light stupor with vivid impressions of a very bizarre experience... ("But, man... I swear there were just hands.... No faces, just hands.... Really freaky.... Hands, poking and talking... And then a giant metal thing came over and sniffed me. I kept real still though and, thank God, it went away.... It was just awful...." "Hey, man, I understand, you were hit on the head.... Things like that happen. You're fine now."—A knowing glance held between visiting friends—"No, really, man, the thing sniffed me and was gonna take a chunk outa my stomach but I lay real still....")

His chest was another story. The right side was clear and sound. A line of ribs was palpated with no apparent deformities or cries of pain. Deep sucks of air were transmitted through my stethoscope like an ocean wave in a conch shell. The right side was fine. The left side was not.

The left side had a large, blue bruise. This discolored area was very tender and if watched carefully seemed to "float."

175

It bobbed alternately with each respiration, up when the chest went down and down when the chest went up. It did not move smoothly or in unison with any other bones. The steering wheel had rammed his ribs violently, cracking them like so much tinder, completely unhinging one entire segment. Now this shard of casting bone kept the man from getting maximum use of what air he managed to inspire. The problem is called a "flail" chest and aptly so, for that section of ribs was indeed flailing around. If things were to normalize, it would require stabilization. But that wasn't all. Even the air that did get in that left lung wasn't going where it was supposed to. It was being routed to strange places. And for bad reasons. There were no breath sounds at all in the upper half of this chest quadrant, a portend of collapsed lung underneath. With its normal path blocked, air was beginning to accumulate in the loose skin surrounding an oozing laceration above the nipple. When I rubbed this gas-filled skin, it felt like silicone. Small soft lumps squished beneath my fingertips. This is called "crepitation," which literally means to "crackle." It comes from an ancient word invented to describe the call of a raven, which, considering the ever-present dark, seemed right in line. This raven crepitus meant that a bronchus had been ruptured and was blowing air out into the chest cavity, where it was finding its way into the skin, there to make crackling sounds like ravens if you rubbed it. A number of things were going to require doing to correct the damage done by that steering wheel.

A quick check of his abdomen found it to be soft and pliant—at last some good news. Seat belts, while generally an extremely good idea, can, in a head-on collision, tear into a strapped stomach, precipitating internal bleeding and a surgical emergency. But his belly was elastic. He didn't wince, even when probed to mid-finger depth.

His legs looked good too. No unnatural angles or exposed spikes of bone. No blue swelling. Only a scratch on either knee where the dash had peeled back skin as he had passed under.

By now the man was coming around. First he began to

moan, then thrash. Waking up is a positive sign for the patient but can make things more difficult for the staff, who must now perform delicate techniques on an agitated and only semi-coherent person. I ordered wrist and ankle restraints just in case.

"Get the thoracic surgeon, please," I called to the unit clerk. It was force of habit. Every wire and charged particle in the entire hospital was dead, including the phone. The desk woman just laughed. A faraway, dark and distant laugh. As far away as the outside world seemed to me now. "Get me a chest tube and let's find a ventilator," I said to a nurse's silhouette. I didn't know if the artificial lungs would work without main power, but the way things were going that night, I strongly doubted it.

Generally I defer major chest procedures to the thoracic surgeon, although a chest tube is not beyond the expertise of a competent Emergency physician. I always like to have him check things anyway, just to be sure. But tonight it didn't matter. Unless someone appeared with two cans and a string I wasn't going to get through to anyone until this issue was long settled, one way or the other.

By the light of a flashlight quartet, a green-towel-wrapped tray was opened and a melange of tubes and metal clamps uncovered. These were spread by a sterile gloved hand, arranged, and made ready for me to jam a plastic hose into my patient's chest. Through that rammed-in pipe I would pull out the unwanted chest air, hoping the deflated lung would reexpand in the process. It all involved the physics of vacuums and air pressure, concepts which I never completely understood but which always seemed to work.

By now the X-rays were back. I put them up to the viewer, then yanked them down in a fit of stupidity and disgust. I would have to read them by flashlight—diagnosis through a keyhole. My circle of light, no larger than the ring a wet glass leaves, moved around the chest film, back and forth. By the time I reached the bottom I had forgotten what was at the top. I went back over everything. I paused at the broken ribs and traced them out. There were six in all, broken in two places each, hence the floating or "flail" phenomenon. The right lung was a bit congested, not out of the ordinary considering that it was probably bruised. The left lung field, however, was very dark. With no lung to block its way, the radiation beam had sped right through. The missing lung cast a small shadow near the bottom of the picture, like a blown-down tent. The dark area, the beam speedway, was where my tube would go and where the rumpled lung tissue would rise to meet it. The abdomen film, thankfully, was normal. A nice, oval stomach bubble resided in the upper right corner. Pockets of air were scattered around the large bowel. I scrutinized the diaphragms and found nothing out of order. Should something of a catastrophic nature have happened in the belly, I might have found collections of air beneath the two thorax dividers. But they were fine—curving, clean, and intact. I was ready to puncture the chest.

I gloved by spotlight and stood to the left of the now nearly awake patient. Again the headlights circled around his chest. I swabbed the immediate area with dark iodine and outlined it with towels. This left a six-inch by six-inch zone of exposed, clean chest through which I would insert my air-collecting tube. "Chest tube, please," I called to a nurse who was to help me. She handed me the long plastic line. I laid it on a sterile towel. "Scalpel." She passed me a cutting knife. I set this down also. "Xylocaine." A syringe full of local anesthetic was next. This I injected around the area between the ribs through which my tube would pass, deep around the nerves that sensed the near bone places. I reached for the scalpel to cut the skin, but never made the incision. I dropped the knife instead. Not because I was clumsy but because I jumped a foot in the air. Something happened to me then that had never happened before, and I hope never will again.

I had told the man that I was going to insert a tube into his chest but I didn't think he had heard me. At the time, he mumbled and swore a bit. I ascribed this to his clearing stupor. But I was wrong. He had understood. And he wanted nothing to do with tubes. Just as I was about to make my first incision, the man bit me. And not just a little poodle nip, the kind you might get from a dog that walks on the end of a shiny leash held by a woman in rhinestone glasses and toreador pants, but a bite like a big ugly dog would give, a dog that lived outside all the time and got kicked a lot. I mean he took a mouthful. Top and bottom. And shook the tar out of my hand like that same dog would do if he got hold of your pants leg. "There," the rabid man said, "that's what I think about your tube."

I looked at my hand. It contained twelve symmetrical holes, each with a rising dot of blood. It was a while before the shock wore off and the pain hit. But when it did, it was sharp and severe. Yet, all things considered, I remained relatively calm. I repressed a strong, sudden desire to leap on top of the bed and stomp the man's face into pudding. Instead, I reproved him vocally. Not one accustomed to cursing, and thus being at somewhat of a disadvantage, I was forced to express my displeasure with a relatively minor shower of epithets, mainly calling into question the ancestry of his parents and wishing eternal evil upon his soul. Minor league insults compared with the motorcycle man, but better suited to my temperament. I considered the pudding option once more, but nixed the idea for good.

What I remember best about the incident, however, was my parting comment as I left to get my hand bandaged. It was something that I would later regret saying, but in a strange way it was something that would give me a measure of satisfaction long after the regret had passed. And, all in all, it was better than pulverizing his face. As I looked at this man's self-satisfied smirk, he came to symbolize all that is wrong with the Emergency Room—the punks, the drunks, the lights, the fights, the hours, the drugs and the creeps, the sore throats, headaches, colds, and always the complaints. "I wasn't seen soon enough"..."I was seen too soon"..."I had too many X-rays"..."I didn't have enough X-rays"..."The bill was too high"..."The bill was too low"...And for this my family spends nights alone? For this I go without sleep? So that some creep can mistake my hand for a ham sandwich? I was trying to save this jerk's life and he bit me. In the calmest voice I could muster, I leaned over and put my head close to his ear. The fellow twisted away, thinking perhaps that I was going to masticate his face in retaliation. But I wasn't. I just wanted to talk. In a voice that only he could hear, I said simply, "I hope you die, clown."

12.

I was at that moment when religious people pray, the weak cry, and the tense take an extra Librium. I was at that moment when the drug-crazed pull out their one special pill, the one given to them by someone at an anti-nuke rally who told them not to take it, or even think about taking it, until they actually saw the mushroom cloud on the horizon, that moment when a person's heart races like the feet of Thumper from the Bambi movie, that moment when jealous lovers shoot guns in blind fury, when men go berserk in the park and tear off their clothes, when soldiers lay down their rifles and walk into the forest or when businessmen leave a note on their windshield and are next seen selling pots on the New Mexico roadside in the company of two Indians and a half-starved dog. In short, I was at my wit's and nerve's end. My mind was alight like a frayed and sparking lamp cord, a firework gone wrong.

A slow winding crank had developed in the back of my head, right where the big neck muscles hook on and pull down on the scalp. It felt as if someone were turning a boat winch and doing it hard enough to lift a huge boat onto a tall pier. My eyes burned like hot coals. My throat was dry and raspy, a testament to the verbal blast I had leveled at the shit-faced geek who chomped on my hand when I tried to save his life. He was the one who had the collapsed lung and, I honestly hoped then, many other things even more obnoxious, like maybe a hole in his heart that was leaking blood just fast enough to make his death certain, but slowly enough for him to know about it, or maybe a weak spot in his main blood artery that was now straining with pressure and would burst at any instant. Or some sort of inoperable brain cancer. Even diabetes would have done, then. My stomach was somewhere past nausea and nearing autolysis. It was long past the point of vomiting.

I was twenty-nine years old, a lunatic whose life I had tried to save had just taken a mouthful of my right hand, it was very late on a Sunday night—a time when people think only bakers and milkmen are awake—I was sitting on a short black stool getting my hand bandaged by a nurse who had to hold a flashlight because the hospital's electric system had gone out, including the backup system, my stomach was a sea of frothing hydrochloric acid, my mental state was such that I was wishing drastic diseases and pox upon my patients and honestly would have rejoiced at the first red bump . . . ("First Case of Smallpox in Five Years," the paper would read. And the more he suffered the better. "Doctor goes berserk! Stomps patient's face! . . . It looked like pudding, witnesses said. Tape at eleven.") I was losing my grip, and fast.

But before I did a swan dive off the edge, strangely enough, I thought about college. I thought about those four years of sacrifice while my friends threw Frisbees, smoked marijuana, and listened to Jimi Hendrix. I remembered seemingly endless days of waking, going to class, coming home and studying, going to bed, tossing for an hour, calling a woman who was superficially my "girlfriend" and having no one answer the phone. I remembered turning down invitiations for weekend trips because I had to study. I remembered walking through the campus library one Saturday night and seeing every student in my Organic Chemistry class, those with whom I was competing for a spot in medical school, all building replica molecules from kits they had sent away for, and then feeling like I had to study all day Sunday just to purge the thought that I didn't even know those kits existed, let alone have any idea where to send for them. I remembered sweating through exams filled with complex chemicals and theorems, all part of the gauntlet through which those people who wished to attend medical school had to run. In my freshman class of 4,000 students, 2,000 answered an entrance questionnaire by saying "Pre-med" was their major. For three and one half years I gave up social, personal, and emotional life to learn about Somebody's Law or So-and-So's Rule and to learn how to make every organic compound found in nature.

I did this for three and one half years, until something snapped. It had snapped then and I was afraid it was going to snap again. I began to fear that maybe I was "snap-prone," that someday the police might have to coax me off a building ledge or persuade me to release the hostages unharmed. I first snapped the night I found my "girlfriend's" apartment dark but with sounds of male and female giggling coming from a couch just below the window. At that moment all the circuits jammed. A cerebral brownout. I went directly home and gathered an armful of my sacrosanct text books, each tome being much revered by either an Oriental physics professor or some pedantic chemistry assistant. I gathered the books into my arms—in itself a superhuman chore—and carried them out to the road, where with demonic pleasure accentuated by hysterical laughter, I skidded them, one by one, across the black, rock-dotted pavement. Then I sat on the curb, as I had done as a boy to count cars, and screamed, loud, long, and hard.

That night I went to bed and slept longer than I had in weeks. When I woke in the morning, the books were scattered far down the street, nearly every page having been tattooed by the zigging geometry of a multitude of tire treads. The bindings were fractured beyond repair. I hoped immense produce trucks had ridden over the larger ones, stopping to back up a time or two. I left those rumpled volumes to posterity and the street sweeper, then drove to campus, where I dropped a Genetics class, took the rest of my courses pass/fail, and, with a roommate, went out to buy a season pass at the municipal golf course. That same day we played thirty-six holes of riotous golf, driving balls all around the course—sometimes five or six per hole, wading into the lake to chase ducks, and consuming large amounts of Coca-Cola. I did not study another minute in college. And I told my "girlfriend" to take a flying leap. Two weeks later I was accepted into medical school.

As white bandages wound round and round my hand and my left shoulder stung with the zing of a tetanus shot, I flashed briefly on medical school. I hit on the memory of long painful nights with many phone calls... "Dr. Seager, we need you again"... "Go to hell."... click.... I remembered only one thing from my internship. That was the very serious thought I had of taking my last paycheck in the form of my beeper and then stomping the electronic bastard into subatomic particles, bits so small that a thousand of them glued together would not have made the tiniest particle known to man.

I thought about all these things while I was getting my hand bandaged, in the dark, very late on a Sunday night, after it had been viciously bitten by a drug-crazed fourth grade drop-out who probably had some horrible festering disease in his chest, for which I was very glad.

By now that river of intestinal acid had reached mid-abdomen and was trying to solder a kink in my small bowel. A strong pain rose, just below my navel. It brought tears to my eyes, then, thankfully, dissipated. My small intestine had held. But the defenses were waning. I knew another attack of the acid brigade could prove fatal. I also knew that I was preparing to fly apart from the force of ten years accumulated nervous energy. I sensed that I was about to splatter all over the far wall like a speeding I.V. bottle, that I was about to disintegrate onto the cold tile floor or self-destruct into hopping bits of Mexican jumping bean dust. I felt as though some super thick amphetamine had been injected directly into my core and was winding its motor for the Great Escape. The pain began again in my stomach; the jags from my hand grew so intense that I could see and taste them. The tendons in my legs were limp and wet. Water ran from the corners of my eyes and the center of my spine. The flashlights grew dark as my head lit out on what gave every indication of being a long and dizzying spin. I could feel every beat of my heart and count each air molecule that was pulled in through hot dry nostrils. The spin accelerated. Then the lights came back on.

With no apology or mention of misbehavior, the lights jacked up and shone, firm and full as though nothing had happened. The blower fan whipped its motor and turned air-moving blades. Soon cool air was nudging out the dark stagnant stuff. Two "Praise the Lord's" came from down the hall. The man with the swollen ankle cheered, as did most of the nurses. And as quickly as they had come, the mob of haunting memories melted like wax in a bonfire. Armegeddon had been postponed. I was back to being just a doctor with a sore hand.

Why do I do what I do? Why do I spend nights and weekends getting bled on, vomited at, and bitten? Why do I stand while others pray at my feet? Why did I give up eight years of my young life to become a doctor? So that I could worry about being sued for everything that I do? For things that mainly are beyond my control? During those eight years I was put into an emotional arrest that caused the breakup of my first marriage, an event that, but for the understanding and the unconditional love of my new wife, Sandy, might have done permanent harm as well. During those eight years that I gave to college and medical school, entire wars were fought and lost, a president was elected and resigned, the Oakland A's won three straight world championships and the Steelers won four Super Bowls, a man walked on the moon. And I didn't see any of it. I bet once on a Met/Oakland World Series game but spent the next thirty hours in labor and delivery and still don't know who won or even whom I made the bet with. Why do I do it? I ask myself that a lot. Why did I give up eight years to get bitten on the hand? Am I a total numbskull? Do I have Cream of Wheat for brains? I am now nearly thirty years old, I have a churning, acid stomach, probably some insidious stress-caused fat deposits in my coronary arteries, and a lingering infection in my hand from some creep with steering wheel marks on his chest. Maybe I fell on my head as a child. Or rolled down a hill and banged my skull on a sharp rock.

I ask why I do it but I always know the answer. I may be a knucklehead, but I'm not stupid. I do it because I like it. Because it's exciting. Because even though most of my patients don't know or care, there are a good number of them walking around today because of me, or riding their motorcycles or shooting heroin or being presidents of banks or doing whatever it is that people do. Then I tell myself to shut up and be thankful.

I hate it, loathe it, despise it, curse it, and will stomp anyone who says otherwise, but I'm hooked. I'm really no better than the "Hey-Man" guys who see snakes crawling up their legs or steal TV sets to buy smack. I'm addicted just like them. I shoot up the E.R. I crave the adrenaline rush from beating back a coma or stopping a bleeding belly. My head and muscles need the charge. I need the juice. I suppose my stomach even needs the acid.

13.

"I can't breathe," said the man from the other room. "When am I going to get that chest tube?" I looked at the nurse as she ripped the last band of tape that held a swarth of dry gauze around my hand. She rolled her eyes. I had a small flair-up of stomach pain but it was weak in comparison to those I had had in the dark. Everything seemed less intense now.

There is a resignation to duty that afflicts soldiers and doctors. You get it either in boot camp or medical school, respectively, experiences, I am told, not all that dissimilar. The country/patient comes first. Do what is right. Don't let personal feelings get in the way. This is a necessary feeling to engender in persons filling these occupations. Surely it is the only thing that makes someone pick up a loaded gun and march toward others similarly outfitted. And it is the only thing that moved my feet back into the accident victim's room to put in that chest tube.

The fellow was now in a lot more distress than when I had left. "Doc," he said with a gasp, "I can't breathe. I need that tube you were talking about." "You mean the chest tube?" I said, reaching for and opening another set of sterile gloves. "Yeah, the chest tube . . . or whatever . . . ." He stopped to take a series of short breaths. "If it will make me breathe better, you can put that tube through my ears. . . . I don't care." Now that reality had set in, his tone was different. This attitude is a distant cousin to "no atheists in a foxhole." All doctors are money-grubbing jerks until you need one. Had I left him to deteriorate further, he would have begun a negotiation session with God. "Please let me breathe, Lord . . . I won't do dope or screw around anymore . . . just get this buzz saw out of my chest. . . ."

"Will you promise not to bite me?" I asked, pushing up a syringe plunger and expressing a speck of local anesthetic through the tip of a needle. I held the plastic cylinder with my left hand and pressed up with a bandaged palm. "Oh yeah," the fellow said, "I'm sorry about that, man." A weak smile followed. "That's okay," I lied, "just as long as your rabies shots are current."

A small lump rose from his chest skin as numbing medicine was reinjected. Then an inch-wide slit was carved with my scalpel. I spread the subcutaneous fat with a clamp and pushed down to bone. Venting a bit of frustration, I closed the clamp and shoved it into his air-filled thoracic cavity. Quickly I jammed a plastic hose in the breech and connected it to a suction device. Air began to filter out and the lung to lift. "Hey, that hurts, man," the patient said as his pulmonary tissue grappled back up his ribs. I smiled and pulled my hands away.

"Now can we get a chest cutter?" I asked the busy ward clerk.

"He's already been called," the woman said smiling, her phone brightly lit with open lines.

"Thank you."

Next I located the partially filled prescription pad for the girl with pneumonia and completed her antibiotic order. I went back to recheck the child and found her sleeping, as were her parents. I explained the discharge instructions to the suddenly awake mother and father. We spoke only briefly. They asked a few questions, which I answered quickly. I was grateful when they accepted the paper leaf without prayer. As I walked back to the nurses' station, they passed by in the hall. The father was carrying his daughter in his arms and lending an elbow to his wife. We exchanged a quick smile.

"Doctor Seager," the clerk said, you are wanted on the phone . . . it's ICU."

"Thanks," I replied and pushed a blinking button on a rack of phone lines. "Hello, this is Doctor Seager."

"Doctor Seager?"

"Yes, what can I do for you?"

"Hold on a minute, sir," a nervous woman said, then dropped the phone on a hard formica counter. I could hear indistinct voices in the background. The only word made out plainly was "Walter."

"Doctor Seager," another voice said, someone else having picked up the fallen phone, "This is Nurse Rothacker, and we need you right away. Your friend Walter is going down the tubes fast. Could you come up and check him?" Before I could answer, she dropped the phone again and ran back to the action.

"I'll be in the ICU," I said, hustling out. In the hallway I passed the sprained ankle man coming back from X-ray. I said that he would have to wait a bit longer for me to read his films because there was an emergency upstairs. I apologized. He said that he understood.

I walked to the elevator, pressed the "Up" button, and waited nervously until the car came. I listened for the front door but it remained closed. No more running fathers with bleeding children. The elevator arrived. I entered and pushed three.

Quickly I was out of the car and into the unit, a menagerie of bleeps, blips, tubes, and tension. Nurses were scurrying from one bed to another like mice on a hot floor, keeping a long row of patients on this side of that fine line. Here was where the fight for life got down and dirty. Here was where our emergency quick hits settled in for the long siege. Here the nurses got to know our momentarily salvaged persons. They fed and bathed them. They talked with the stunned families. Their patients died as friends. I realized then that Emergency Room anonymity was not without merit. At least when people died down there they did so as strangers.

Most of the nurses were clustered around the bed of Walter T., the bridegroom who had prepared for the coming ceremony by filling his lungs with water and choking off his brain. You could hear his labored, wet breathing from out in the hall.

Walter looked bad even for him. His yellow egg body had swollen further and deepened in hue, taking on a green cast, like moldy mustard. As any eighth grade art student will tell you, when you mix yellow, the pigment deposited in Walter's skin, with blue, the tone produced by Walter's general lack of oxygen, you get green. And Walter was green.

His breathing was shallow and rapid, more rapid than I had ever seen anyone breathe. He sounded like a very adept tap dancer performing a difficult passage. His mouth emitted short crisp chirps in a regular speedy cadence. He had lapsed back into coma. Things looked grim.

I knew that the standard measures of treatment might help but in themselves would not be enough. I needed something quick, dramatic, and immediate. I called for a phlebotomy set.

In a last-ditch effort to relieve fluid pressure on Walter's heart, thus allowing it to more efficiently pump blood with its disease-ravaged muscle fibers, I was forced to take the direct route. With no place left inside, the fluid would have to come outside. In the aptly named "Dark Ages," a common medical practice was to bleed sick persons. This was thought to let out bad humors and return a person to spiritual and physical balance. Needless to say, the majority of people were not helped in the slightest and a good many were grievously harmed. "God's will" no doubt was blamed for many an iatrogenic death. Then why, you may wonder, wasn't the practice abandoned when even the dullest clayhead or sodridden serf could see that bleeding was a waste of time and that no one ever got better? Because, unfortunately, some people did get better. Not because "evil sap" was tapped but because removing blood, which is fluid, relieved pressure on failing hearts. Thus, tenth-century persons who suffered with congestive heart failure and pulmonary edema benefited from these priestly blood baths. Everybody got bled because of it.

Had I owned a Hamlet suit, I would have put it on. Sucking blood into glass bottles was better suited for sackcloth, capes, and a chanting monk. "Light the incense, Nurse," I said, then asked if anyone could recite Chaucer. The phlebotomy apparatus, a vacuum bottle with needle and hose, is made to siphon blood. A modern-day leech and bowl. It is the same sort of setup used when a person gives blood. And Walter T. was about to give blood.

Like Dracula near sunrise, I scavenged earnestly for a vein. Finding a good thick one, I quickly plunged my needle in. As if driven by its own desire, the metal spire struck red oil and a geyser shot into the bottle. I drew off two units, then called off my minions. I had bled my patient. And, by God, and Thomas Aquinas, he got better.

Walter stopped puffing like a hummingbird's wing and began to take respirations that could be counted. His heartbeat dropped from the stratosphere to a regular, although slightly rapid rate. For the moment his heart beat joyfully. But I knew that even the slightest untoward event would plunge it back into distress. Things were very tight. I had to put the wedding into fast forward.

I left the bedside and headed for the ICU waiting room, which consisted of a couch and television set stuck in a corner of the hall. Nervous families sit there watching doctors come and go, trying to read prognoses from the expression on their physician's face. I found Sumi on the couch.

She saw me coming and asked if Walter was dead. I said no, but remarked that this was merely a judgment call. I said that things were going to have to be moved up. Walter simply had no time to spare. If there was to be a wedding it would have to be very soon. "Could we do it here?" the woman asked politely. "Of course," I replied. And that was enough. She excused herself to make a phone call. In twenty minutes a priest appeared.

I made hasty plans with the ICU staff. A nurse was dispatched downstairs and returned with a roll of blue crepe paper. "Stole it from the bulletin board," she said matter-of-factly. Walter's bed sheets and gown were changed in deference to the occasion, while the bunting was strung along a horseshoe curtain rail that swung around the bed. It looked like a long, flat, azure snake had taken refuge in the drape rods.

As if on cue, Walter roused from his liver coma and mumbled something vaguely coherent. A nurse leaned over and nodded. He spoke again. She seemed to understand. The

191

woman walked away and returned with a vase and one wilted flower. A patient in the next bed had expired during the day and one of her flowers had been fished from the trash. The drooping daisy perked up slightly when dipped in fresh water and placed in a paper cup on Walter's nightstand.

Then the priest rushed in, blurry-eyed but ready. He understood the gravity of the situation, he said, and was happy to be of service. I took him aside anyway and explained about the seriousness of Walter's condition, about his paper-thin heart muscle and the Atlantic Ocean running in his veins. We agreed to skip any frivolities and get right to the meat. Everyone took their places. With myself on Walter's right and a string of attendant staff to his left, we watched as Sumi entered. She was on the arm of an orderly. They walked in step to the bedside, to the tune of Walter's cardiac monitor. The sick man nodded imperceptibly and smiled when his bride appeared around the curtain. They shared a look that transcended thirty years. For just a candle flicker they were back in the Pacific. Walter the patient and she his nurse. As before, clouds of doom were gathered outside. Only this time the clouds would not be driven away. This time they would bring black rain, engulf Walter, and carry him away.

"Are we ready?" the priest asked around to the assembled faces. We all nodded our heads. "Dearly beloved..." the man begin in a firm voice that carried to every ear and heart in the room.

Walter listened intently to a very brief greeting and invocation, then suddenly became agitated. He muttered something in a sharp, quick voice. "What is it, Walter?" one of the nurses asked. Two others bent closer to hear. "I don't understand, Walter, what do you want?" one of them said.

"It's the flower," Sumi said quietly.

"The flower?" I said.

"Yes. He wants me to have the flower. Every bride needs a bouquet," she said correctly. And she got it. A nurse quickly extracted the bud from its container and gently passed it to the tiny lady. Sumi held the stem lightly as does one made

192

to handle flowers. But the delay and the excitement had begun to tell on Walter. I watched as his chest movements quickened and his eyes glassed slightly.

By then Sumi had repeated her vows. "I do," she said in an Asian accent that must have been the same as when Walter first heard it 10,000 miles across the ocean. "I do," she said a second time, and everyone smiled. "And do you Walter, take Sumi . . . " was as far as things got before Walter went really bad again. In a flash, like a wave washing over a beach, blue and green crept over the sick man's face. The hummingbird breathing began anew. "He's going to die before we finish," one of the nurses said and then wished that she hadn't. There was general commotion around the bed, hands reaching for I.V. lines, fingers checking pulses. Sumi took one step back and said nothing. She did not cry nor did she comment. She was marrying Walter because she loved him, because he wanted to marry her. She was concerned only about Walter, not about being a beneficiary. If Walter died in mid-ceremony, so be it. At least they had been together.

I reached into a back pocket and produced a large medicine-filled syringe. I had suspected Walter might fade so I had prepared it in advance. I knelt at his side, took his I.V. line in hand, and injected the big dose of diuretic medication. I needed only five seconds, just time for an "I do" and a kiss. The drug took a minute or so to circulate but then did its job. Walter's color blanched, returning him to his natural yellow. He breathed more slowly. His eyes reopened. He was teetering on a fence but, for the moment, leaning toward life. I made a circling gesture with my index finger and the priest responded. He tore through the groom's vows like a runaway train. At the end, beads of sweat glowed on his forehead. He leaned in for Walter's response. "I do," the dying man croaked, and we all heard it. "By the power vested in me by this state," a much relieved cleric said, "I now pronounce you man and wife." "You may now kiss the bride," he said to Walter, then looked at Sumi. She edged closer to the bed, touched both lips to her husband's cheek, and said something in Japanese that we did not understand. But Walter understood. He turned toward his bride and smiled for the last time in his life.

I shook Walter's sagging hand and kissed Sumi, who now allowed herself a smile also. The nurses all hugged the diminutive woman, having to bend down to do so. No one had a dry eye. It was a moment common to all weddings, that short ethereal instant when life seems worthwhile, despite the circumstance, and things are right with God. Then we left the newlyweds alone. It was their time to spend together. Their honeymoon. Once again they were far away. In each other's arms. With strange and forboding noises in the background.

As we opened the curtains to leave, we saw the day shift coming on. They were all clustered in the window and staring. None had dared enter or speak. They remained silent as the wedding party passed on their way to the waiting room. One of the nurses wiped a tear from her eye.

"I always cry at weddings," she said to the startled newcomers.

I looked at the clock. It was 5:30. My body felt like noon. But if it was 5:30, why was the day crew here? Then I remembered the dark and realized that the electric clocks had stopped too. It was really 7:00 A.M., and the night, indeed the entire weekend, was over. A wave of reprieve swept over me. I felt like a prisoner granted clemency, as if someone had lifted a great sandbag off my shoulders. Now I smiled.

After she had spoken with Walter, I escorted Sumi out to the waiting room and spoke with her for a moment. Then a nurse beckoned to me from the unit door. I went back in and pronounced Walter dead. I told Sumi. Again she showed no emotion. There was no need. She was Walter's wife, and she knew that she had given her husband the only true happiness he had ever known. Their life together had started in a hospital and ended in a hospital. He had been hers during those heady days in the South Pacific and hers when he died. This was not reason to cry. There was comfort in that.

194

After a minute Sumi stood. She picked up the wilted flower that had been her bouquet and walked slowly to the elevator. When a car came she got in. Never once did she look back. The doors slid closed and she was gone.

I spoke briefly with the ICU nurses before I left, thanking them for their time and help. In turn, they reminded me that the pharmacist had survived his operation, the one who got the blood, just as the young man had who did without. They said both patients were stable and well on the way to recovery. In two weeks my friend would leave the hospital and in a month return to work. The youthful thief also would leave the hospital, wearing the same threadbare tennis shoes with which he had crept up on our pharmacist. After his sutures were removed, neither I, the pharmacist, or his surgeon ever heard from him again. In a month the last of an elliptical row of scars would fall from my hand and there would be no more pain.

"Your ankle is only sprained," I said to the long-suffering man with the blue bulge on his foot. "The X-rays were normal." I laid an icebag over the swelling. "You will, however, need to walk with crutches for a week and see your doctor on Wednesday for a recheck." During all of this the man nodded but I could tell he needed more. "I'm sorry you had to wait so long," I said sincerely, "but the lights went out and we had a wedding in the Intensive Care Unit." The man looked at me. At his ankle. At the ceiling. And at the lights. "I understand," he said.